Springhouse Review for
PSYCHIATRIC & MENTAL HEALTH NURSING CERTIFICATION

THIRD EDITION

Springhouse Review for
PSYCHIATRIC & MENTAL HEALTH NURSING CERTIFICATION

THIRD EDITION

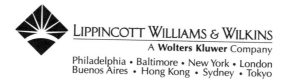

LIPPINCOTT WILLIAMS & WILKINS
A **Wolters Kluwer** Company
Philadelphia • Baltimore • New York • London
Buenos Aires • Hong Kong • Sydney • Tokyo

STAFF

Publisher
Judith A. Schilling McCann, RN, MSN

Editorial Director
David Moreau

Clinical Director
Joan M. Robinson, RN, MSN, CCRN

Senior Art Director
Arlene Putterman

Clinical Editor
Joanne M. Bartelmo, RN, MSN

Editors
Julie Munden (senior editor), Liz Schaeffer (associate editor), Laura Marshfield, Carol Munson

Copy Editors
Peggy Williams (copy supervisor), Kimberly Bilotta, Thomas DeZego, Shana Harrington, Elizabeth Mooney, Marcia Ryan, Pamela Wingrod

Designers
Debra Moloshok (book design), ON-TRAK Graphics, Inc., Donna S. Morris

Electronic Production Services
Diane Paluba (manager), Joyce Rossi Biletz

Manufacturing
Patricia K. Dorshaw (manager), Beth Janae Orr

Editorial Assistants
Danielle J. Barsky, Beverly Lane, Linda Ruhf

Indexer
Karen Comerford

Printed in the United States of America.

SRPSY3 – D N O S A J J M A M
04 03 02   10 9 8 7 6 5 4 3 2 1

Library of Congress Cataloging-in-Publication Data

Springhouse review for psychiatric and mental health nursing certification. — 3rd ed.
    p. ; cm.
  Rev. ed. of: American nursing review for psychiatric and mental health nursing certification/Nancy Randolph. 2nd ed. c1998.
  Includes bibliographical references and index.
Psychiatric nursing — Outlines, syllabi, etc. 2. Psychiatric nursing Examinations, questions, etc. I. Title: Review for psychiatric and mental health nursing certification. II. Randolph, Nancy. American nursing review for psychiatric and mental health nursing certification. III. Lippincott Williams & Wilkins.
  [DNLM: 1. Mental Disorders — nursing — Examination Questions. 2. Mental Disorders — nursing — Outlines. 3. Psychiatric Nursing — methods — Examination Questions. 4. Psychiatric Nursing — methods — Outlines. WY 18.2 S7698 2002]
RC440 .R33 2002
610.73'68'076 — dc21
ISBN 1-58255-173-1 (alk. paper)
               2001057632

Contents

Contributors

Colleen C. Burgess, RN, MSN, APRN, BC-CS, NCSAC
Nursing Instructor
Carolinas College of Health Sciences
Charlotte, N.C.

Linda Carman Copel, RN, PhD, CS, DAPA
Associate Professor
Villanova (Pa.) University

Claire Burke Draucker, RN, PhD, CS
Professor and Director, Graduate Program in Psychiatric Mental Health Nursing
Kent State (Ohio) University

Charlene K. Eshleman, RN, CS
Psychiatric Clinical Nurse Specialist
Private Practice and Lancaster Regional Medical Center
Columbia, Pa. and Lancaster, Pa.

Anne H. Fishel, RN, PhD, CS
Professor and Chair Academic Division II
University of North Carolina
Chapel Hill

Connie S. Heflin, RN, MSN
Professor of Nursing
Paducah (Ky.) Community College

Kathleen J. Hudson, RN, MSN
Nursing Instructor
Illinois Eastern Community Colleges — WVC Campus
Mt. Carmel

Karla Jones, RN, MS
Nursing Instructor
Treasure Valley Community College
Ontario, Ore.

May E. Phillips, RN, PhD
Independent Consultant
Gettysburg, Pa.

Barbara C. Rynerson, RN, MS, CS
Therapist and Consultant
Magellan Behavioral Health
Raleigh, N.C.

Foreword

In today's fast-paced arena of psychiatric and mental health nursing, expert knowledge helps maintain clinical excellence in any practice setting. Certification in psychiatric and mental health nursing provides professional recognition of a nurse's high achievement of specialty knowledge and superior nursing practice. It's a signal to both professional peers and the public of a nurse's advanced qualifications in psychiatric and mental health nursing practice.

Nurses who take the American Nurses Association's (ANA's) certification examination must demonstrate superior knowledge of psychiatric and mental health nursing and the ability to apply that knowledge to a wide variety of psychiatric clients in varied health care settings. To pass the test, the nurse must resharpen test-taking skills and develop new strategies for answering test questions that differ in style from those the nurse may remember appearing on the state boards.

Springhouse Review for Psychiatric and Mental Health Nursing Certification, Third Edition, helps the nurse prepare for ANA's Psychiatric and Mental Health Nursing Certification Examination. Each chapter has been thoroughly reviewed and updated to include the latest information on psychiatric disorders and treatments. The easy-to-follow outline format contains all of the elements needed to:
- understand how the examination is developed and scored.
- complete a thorough review of psychiatric nursing concepts, theories, and practices.
- evaluate readiness to take the actual examination.

Chapter 1 describes the eligibility requirements for taking the test and reviews the examination blueprint. Knowing what's likely to be on the examination is fundamental to knowing what to study. To give the nurse a framework for building self-confidence, the chapter also offers proven test-taking strategies, analyzes the structure of test questions, and provides hints for selecting the correct answer.

Chapter 2 reviews concepts central to understanding basic human emotional responses from anxiety to anger to grief. Chapter 3 explores human development. Chapter 4 reviews the ever-expanding settings, roles, and scope of psychiatric and mental health nursing practice. Chapter 5 focuses on theoretical models of human behavior. Chapter 6 reviews the techniques of gathering, manipulating, and reporting research data, an important component of advanced practice.

Chapter 7 covers therapeutic communication, one of the primary tools of psychiatric and mental health nursing practice. Chapter 8 explains the essential legal aspects of nursing practice, such as informed consent, confinement, and clients' rights.

Chapters 9 through 17 cover the major psychiatric disorders seen by psychiatric and mental health nurses, such as anxiety disorders, mood disorders, and personality disorders. The text reviews causes, signs and symptoms, possible nursing diagnoses, and nursing interventions. Additionally, the text presents relevant diagnostic criteria from the *Diagnostic and Statistical Manual of Mental Disorders*, 4th Edition, Text Revision (perhaps better known by the abbreviated name, *DSM-IV-TR*). Each of these chapters also includes a clinical situation (case study) based on one of the disorders discussed in that chapter. Organized around the nursing process, the clinical situation examines the client's health problems through the phases of assessment, diagnosis, planning, implementation, and evaluation. Rationales for each nursing action (in italic type) give the reader a complete foundation for planning nursing care.

Chapter 18 reviews the individual, group, and rehabilitative therapies commonly used to treat psychiatric disorders, including their purpose, indications for use, and nursing implications.

Chapter 19 covers the major drug groups used in psychiatric treatment: antipsychotic agents, antiparkinsonian agents, tricyclic antidepressants, monoamine oxidase inhibitors, antimanic agents, benzodiazepines, and sedative-hypnotic agents. For each group, the text presents indications, mechanism of action, pharmacokinetics, adverse effects, contraindications, and nursing implications. Tables for each group provide information about specific pharmaceutical products.

New to this third edition are review questions that appear at the end of chapters 2 through 19. These questions test your knowledge of the concepts covered in each chapter and provide you with instant feedback.

The posttest, written in the same format used on the actual examination, covers all study areas that appear in the certification blueprint. Correct answers and rationales follow, along with a diagnostic profile, to give the nurse a reliable indication of which areas require further study.

Two appendices provide information for additional preparation: the ANA's standards of psychiatric and mental health nursing practice and the NANDA-approved taxonomy of nursing diagnoses, revised in 2000. Selected references offer opportunities for further study and research, and the index serves as a handy guide when trying to locate a topic quickly.

Springhouse Review for Psychiatric and Mental Health Nursing Certification, Third Edition, is a comprehensive resource that contains all the information a nurse needs to prepare successfully for the psychiatric and mental health nursing certification examination. I hope this book helps you in your quest for certification and that you use it as a reference in your practice for many years.

Rick Zoucha, APRN, BC, CTN, DNSc
Associate Professor
Duquesne University
School of Nursing
Pittsburgh

Certification examination

In 1973, the American Nurses Association (ANA) established a certification program in psychiatric and mental health nursing to recognize the expert knowledge and practice of psychiatric nurses. It's the second largest of all ANA certification programs.

The ANA offers three examinations for psychiatric nursing certification: a basic psychiatric and mental health nurse examination, a clinical specialist examination for adult psychiatric and mental health nursing, and a clinical specialist examination for child and adolescent psychiatric and mental health nursing. Administered by the American Nurses Credentialing Center (ANCC) each June and October in cities throughout the United States and its territories, the examinations are given in the morning and last about 3 hours.

Eligibility and application

The ANCC establishes criteria for eligibility to take the examination. Requirements for the basic examination differ from those for the clinical specialist examinations. Because requirements can change, candidates should obtain the latest criteria before applying for certification. (See *Certification eligibility requirements*, page 2.)

Once you have decided to prepare for the examination, you may want to obtain the certification catalog by writing to the American Nurses Credentialing Center, 600 Maryland Ave., S.W., Suite 100 West, Washington, DC 20024; by calling toll free, 1-800-284-2378; or by visiting the ANCC Web site at *www.nursingworld.org*. This catalog provides all the information you'll need to apply.

Pay careful attention to all steps in the application process. Failure to complete a step correctly may make you ineligible to take the examination on the date you had planned. All applicants must pay a nonrefundable application fee and an examination fee, set each year by the credentialing center.

Certification eligibility requirements

The American Nurses Credentialing Center's eligibility criteria for certification in psychiatric and mental health nursing, effective December 31, 2001, are listed below. Note that the requirements for the basic examination differ from those of the specialist examinations.

Criteria for a psychiatric and mental health nurse

By the time of application, you must:
- hold an active registered nurse license in the United States or its territories
- have practiced as a licensed RN for 2 years full-time in the U.S. or its territories and have a minimum of 2,000 hours of clinical practice within the past 3 years (nursing faculty may apply up to 500 hours of teaching or clinical supervision in the specialty area of practice toward the practice requirement; students may apply up to 500 hours of time spent in an academic program of nursing study toward the clinical practice requirement)
- be involved in direct psychiatric and mental health nursing practice for an average of 8 hours per week (direct patient care is interaction involving the nursing process [assessment, planning, treatment, coordination, management, consultation, evaluation, and revision of a care plan] for individuals, families, and communities; the interaction may be through face-to-face contact with the patient or via electronic communications, such as the Internet, telephone, tele-health, and video-conferencing care technologies)
- have access to clinical consultation or supervision
- submit a reference from a nurse colleague on Form B, obtained from the American Nurses Association (if the nurse isn't from your place of employment, you must submit an additional reference from a nonnurse mental health colleague from your place of employment on Form C; this reference is based on any arrangement that allows psychiatric and mental health nurses to discuss their work in an ongoing way with an experienced mental health colleague)
- have had 30 contact hours of continuing education applicable to the specialty area in the past 3 years.

Criteria for a clinical specialist in adult or child and adolescent psychiatric and mental health nursing

By the time of application, you must hold a master's degree or higher in nursing with a university-identified major in psychiatric and mental health nursing. (A university-identified major is one that's listed in the university course catalog and contains specific psychiatric and mental health nursing didactic and clinical experiences.) Advanced practice registered nurses seeking certification as clinical specialists can apply for initial certification as soon as they graduate, provided they have received 500 hours of supervised clinical practicum within their academic program.

Candidates who don't have a master's degree or higher in psychiatric and mental health nursing must meet the following criteria:
- hold a master's degree or higher in nursing
- have a minimum of 18 graduate or postgraduate academic credits in psychiatric and mental health theory (at least 9 of these 18 credits must contain didactic and clinical experience specific to psychiatric and mental health nursing theory; core courses in nursing theory, nursing research, and thesis hours will not be accepted as part of this 9-credit requirement; a maximum of 9 of the 18 graduate or postgraduate credits may be in courses containing didactic and clinical experiences specific to psychiatric and mental health theory [for example, courses in counseling and psychology])
- have supervised clinical training at the graduate or postgraduate level in two psychotherapeutic treatment modalities.

Certification test plan

After establishing your eligibility, the credentialing center will mail you a handbook that contains the current examination blueprint, or test plan. This plan delineates the test content and the ratio (weighting) of each content area for that particular test. Information about the test plan, especially its content, can provide considerable guidance in helping you organize your study plan.

The basic examination in psychiatric and mental health nursing includes these domains of practice:

* concepts and theories — nursing process, therapeutic relationship, conceptual frameworks and nursing models, developmental and psychological theories, group dynamics theories, health promotion and disease prevention
* psychopathology — chemical dependency, violence, and disorders of mood, anxiety, organic, personality, and thought
* treatment modalities — milieu therapy; individual, group, and family therapy; crisis management; behavioral therapies; biological therapies
* professional issues and trends — ethical and legal issues, quality improvement, management, political and social issues, standards of practice, education, consultation-liaison and collaboration issues, research, and cultural and ethnic issues.

According to the certification catalog, all parts of the nursing process and interdisciplinary collaboration will be represented in examination items within the appropriate content category.

The Board on Certification for Psychiatric and Mental Health Nursing Practice develops the certification examination. This test objectively evaluates knowledge, comprehension, and application of psychiatric nursing theory and practice in patient care. For each test, the committee defines the content areas as well as the emphasis placed on each area. The Commission on Certification (COC) has approved converting the clinical nurse specialist examinations to a computer-based format after May 2001.

Certified psychiatric and mental health nurses from around the country contribute questions for each examination. The test-development committee reviews each test item for accuracy, readability, and relevance to the test plan. Sample questions approved by the committee are compiled into an examination that will be used on the next test date.

Each test contains 175 multiple-choice questions, of which 150 are scored questions and 25 are nonscored (pretest) questions. Pretest questions aren't differentiated from scored questions. Any answers left blank (unanswered) will be scored as incorrect. Candidates have 4 hours to complete the test.

Test results are mailed to all candidates about 6 to 8 weeks after the examination. To protect the privacy of candidates, no results are released early or over the telephone.

Preparing for the certification examination

To ensure success on the examination, you must know how to analyze questions and use specific strategies to help you select the best response. Readiness for taking the test involves three areas of preparation: intellectual, physical, and emotional.

Intellectual preparation includes a complete review of all the subjects that will be covered on the test. This book provides you with an organized source for that review. Supplement its use with other sources, such as current medical and nursing literature, particularly if the subject isn't one you deal with every day in your practice. If you take a review course, pay special attention to unfamiliar material being discussed, and be sure to ask the instructor for clarification when necessary. You also may want to discuss topics covered in the review course with other participants or perhaps organize a study group to review difficult material after the course is over.

Finally, take the posttest included in this book; then review the correct answers and analyze your performance by completing the accompanying diagnostic profile. The posttest will provide questions from all content areas of the certification examination, and the diagnostic profile will help you pinpoint the reasons for incorrect answers, thereby suggesting areas for further study to help you avoid repeating these mistakes on the actual test.

Physical preparation for the examination may seem obvious, but many candidates ignore its importance. Staying up all night before the test to cram last-minute information is an obvious mistake. Sound physical preparation also involves applying for the test well in advance and securing all the necessary documents to ensure your eligibility. Keep your test permit in a safe place, and remember to take it with you to the examination. If you live near the examination site, visit it in advance to gauge travel time and familiarize yourself with parking facilities. Nothing can affect your performance more adversely than arriving late in a state of high anxiety. Make overnight reservations early if you have to travel a long distance. Staying close to the test location will promote a good night's sleep and prompt arrival. If you're sensitive to room temperature, plan to take a sweater that's easy to put on or remove. Take mints or hard candy to relieve a dry mouth. Finally, eat a light but nourishing breakfast that will give you energy for performing at an optimum level.

Emotional preparation markedly influences test performance. Be confident. Think positively. Look at the examination as a way of demonstrating your mastery of the subject matter. After all, you have been practicing psychiatric nursing for many years. You have a wealth of knowledge about most of the test content. You have taken standardized tests before, the most memorable being the NCLEX-RN (state boards). Everyone is anxious before an important examination. The feeling is normal, even beneficial. All psychiatric nurses know that mild anxiety keeps you alert, motivates you to study, and helps you to concentrate. However, you also know that too little or too much anxiety can affect performance. Think about past experiences when you have been anxious during a test. If you recall being too anxious, now is the time to learn some simple relaxation exercises, such as rhythmic breathing and progressive muscle relaxation. Guided imagery, such as imagining yourself successfully answering all the questions on the test, can be helpful. Remind yourself of those relaxation techniques that worked in the past. They can work again. During the test, avoid becoming distracted by others who may be exhibiting anxious behavior. Concentrate on the test in front of you, and keep your feelings under control. Positive feelings will help you relax and keep your confidence high. Don't be bothered by people who seem to have finished the test early. Tell yourself that they have just given up and probably didn't complete the examination.

Test-taking strategies

You can improve your chances of passing standardized multiple-choice examinations by using techniques that have proved successful for others. These techniques include knowing how timed examinations are administered, understanding all the parts of a test question, and taking specific steps to ensure that you have selected the correct answer.

Time management becomes crucial when taking a standardized test because the candidate receives no credit for unanswered questions. Consequently, you should try to pace yourself to finish the test on time. Remember, you'll have about 1 minute to answer each question. Don't spend too much time on any one question. Keep in mind that you won't be penalized for guessing. If you have no idea of the correct answer, select any option; you still have a 25% chance of being correct.

All questions on the certification examination have been carefully crafted and pretested to ensure readability and uniformity. Understanding the components of a question can help you analyze what the question is asking, a strategy which will increase the likelihood that you will respond correctly. The diagram on the next page shows the parts of a multiple-choice question. Note how clearly the question is written, with no unnecessary words. Each option in the answer is relatively uniform in length. (See *Parts of a test question,* page 6.)

Read every question carefully. If a description of a clinical situation precedes the question, study the information given. Watch for key words— such as *most, first, best,* and *except.* They're important guides to which option you should select. For example, if a question reads, "Which of the following nursing actions should the nurse perform first?" you may find that all the listed options are appropriate for the patient's condition, but only one of them clearly takes precedence over the others.

As you read the question, try to anticipate the correct answer. Look at the options to see if your answer is listed. If so, it's probably the correct one.

If you don't see your expected answer in the options, read all the options again before you select one. If you select an option before reading all

Parts of a test question

Multiple-choice test questions on the certification examination are constructed according to strict psychometric standards. As shown below, each question has a stem and four options — a key (correct answer) and three distracters (incorrect answers). A brief clinical situation, or case study, usually precedes the questions.

1. You're approached by a 46-year-old patient who appears disheveled and is wearing a full hockey outfit. Moving close to your face, he says, with no affect, "Let's make love."

Stem — The most likely inference for you to make about this patient is that he:

Options

- ○ is trying to embarrass you. —————————————————— Distracter
- ○ is asking you to relate with him. —————————————————— Key (correct answer)
- ○ has unmet psychosexual needs. —————————————————— Distracter
- ○ probably dislikes women. —————————————————— Distracter

of them, you'll deny yourself the opportunity to evaluate all the choices. Try to find an option that most closely resembles the one you thought would be correct. If you don't find one, look for the best option available. Remember, you're looking for the best answer among those given. It may not be what you think is the best response, but it's all you have to work with.

For some questions, you may see two options that seem correct and you can't decide between them. Look at them again. There has to be a difference. Read the question again. You may discover something that you didn't see before that will help you make a selection. If not, and you still can't choose, make an educated guess, and place a light mark by the question so you can return to it later.

Despite thorough preparation, you may not know the answer to some questions. Relax. Remember that you're an expert practitioner; you possess a wealth of information. Think of patient cases that you have had, and recall information about them that you can apply to the question. Tell yourself the principle involved, and recall what you know about applying that principle to practice situations. At the very least, this will help you eliminate some of the options that are probably wrong. Now you may have narrowed the selections to perhaps two options. This should make your choice easier.

Taking the certification examination shows your confidence in your knowledge about psychiatric nursing. Following an organized study program, such as the one provided in the following pages, will help ensure that you're fully prepared to take the test.

Fundamental concepts

❖ **Anxiety**

■ Anxiety is a universal, subjective feeling of vague, generalized apprehension

■ This emotion is crucial to human survival, yet excessively high levels of anxiety can interfere with one's ability to maintain health

■ Four theories of anxiety hold special importance for psychiatric and mental health nursing

◆ In the late 19th century, with his *psychodynamic theory*, Freud first discussed a psychological basis for anxiety

▶ Anxiety signals the ego of an emerging unconscious impulse

▶ Anxiety is a key emotion of the ego, indicating hidden psychological conflicts

◆ According to the *learned theory*, which was first proposed about 1977 by Bandura and others, anxiety is a learned response to an unpleasant stimulus

▶ Avoiding the unpleasant stimulus reduces anxiety

▶ The person ultimately learns to avoid unpleasant stimuli

◆ The *biochemical theory*, which evolved from the work of many theorists from 1977 to 1980, proposes that high anxiety levels correlate with increases in heart rate, blood lactase levels, and oxygen use during moderate exercise

▶ These changes increase midbrain activity which, in turn, releases norepinephrine

▶ Increased norepinephrine in humans increases anxiety

▶ Gamma-aminobutyric acid (GABA), a neurotransmitter that normally inhibits anxiety, functions abnormally and doesn't stop (or reduce) the anxiety

◆ In 1986, Marks formulated the *genetic theory*

▶ All organisms, including humans, are selectively bred for defensive behavior

▶ Autonomic susceptibility to threats is genetically determined

■ Anxiety has two categories

◆ *Acute anxiety (state anxiety)* is transient apprehension that fluctuates in intensity and usually relates to a specific situation or occurrence; it's an intense physical and psychological episode that occurs without warning and causes a sense of impending doom

◆ *Chronic anxiety (trait anxiety)* is a permanent characteristic marked by strong, frequent bouts of anxiety from precipitating stressors, such as threats to self-esteem or physical safety; it's a fixed part of one's personality that's manifested by nervousness, insomnia, and continual irritability

■ An individual can experience four levels of anxiety

◆ *Mild anxiety* is a normal state of tension characterized by alertness; enhanced concentration and perception; a sharpened ability to think, reason, and learn; and a high level of motivation resulting in organized and focused behavior

◆ *Moderate anxiety* narrows one's focus, causing the individual to ignore or block out selective parts of what caused the anxiety level to rise; characteristics include selective attention, reduced perception and concentration, diminished thinking and problem-solving abilities, and behavior that focuses on the immediate interest

◆ *Severe anxiety* markedly reduces one's ability to cope with life's events because the individual focuses totally on a specific event to the exclusion of everything else; characteristics include markedly narrowed perception, loss of concentration, internally directed attention to relieve distress from the anxiety, and severely reduced thinking, reasoning, and problem-solving abilities

◆ *Panic anxiety* is an extreme maladaptive response to stress characterized by greatly impaired perception; complete disorganization of the personality; inability to reason, solve problems, or think rationally; and complete inability to function safely without help

■ Anxiety is manifested psychologically, physically, and cognitively

◆ *Psychological symptoms* include a feeling of impending doom, decreased perception, loss of control, tension, nervousness, and withdrawal from others

◆ *Physical symptoms* include syncope; shortness of breath; heart palpitations; a "lump" in the throat; sweating, especially in the palms; and nausea or "butterflies"

◆ *Cognitive symptoms* include loss of attention, reduced ability to solve problems, impaired concentration, inability to make decisions, and reduced work productivity

■ Health screening for anxiety includes assessing the patient's physical, psychological, and social background; the patient is assisted in linking the feeling of anxiety with the behavior that manifests

❖ **Stress**

■ Stress is any biopsychosocial external or internal experience that one views as demanding, challenging, and threatening

■ Stress is a dynamic process that contributes to personal survival and growth or behavioral dysfunction and death

■ In 1950, Selye advanced the study of stress theory by articulating the generalized adaptation syndrome

◆ Selye identified three stages of stress response in humans
 ▶ The *alarm reaction* mobilizes the body's defense resources against a real or perceived threat
 ▶ The body begins to adapt through increased resistance to the stressor
 ▶ *Exhaustion* occurs when the body's resources are depleted and can't resist the stressor
◆ These responses, based on Selye's postulates, may be adaptive or maladaptive
◆ One's ability to recognize stress is crucial to the success of stress management

■ Stressors usually occur in groups over time; the number of stressors and the time they occur influence one's ability to cope with them
◆ In 1967, Holmes and Rahe developed a list of "stressful life events"; ranked according to the coping behavior required of a person, the top 10 stressors are death of a spouse, divorce, marital separation, jail term, death of a close family member, personal injury or illness, marriage, termination from employment, marital reconciliation, and retirement
◆ More recent studies by Cassel, Cobb, and Caplan suggest that the magnitude of life changes resulting from the stressor is more important than the stressor itself
◆ Other research shows that the dissatisfactions with and problems of everyday life accumulate over time and ultimately have a greater effect on mental well-being than specific stressors

■ Human response to stress depends on one's perception of the stressor, available coping resources, intellectual and emotional states, and sense of well-being
◆ How a person responds to stress can be affected by physiologic, psychological, and sociocultural factors
 ▶ Physiologic factors include one's genetic makeup, nutritional status, and overall health
 ▶ Psychological factors include innate intelligence, self-esteem, sense of self-control, and morale
 ▶ Sociocultural factors include one's age, educational preparation, occupation, and economic status
◆ The psychophysiologic signs of stress are the same as those of anxiety (see "Anxiety," pages 7 and 8)

■ Health education and individual patient teaching can mitigate the effects of stress; commonly used stress management techniques include meditation, biofeedback, relaxation exercises (such as progressive muscle relaxation [PMR]), stress-inoculation training, and complementary therapies (such as yoga and the herb kava-kava)

❖ Anger

- One of the primary human emotions, anger is a feeling of displeasure that occurs when one perceives a threat; the resulting tension must be released to avoid physical or psychological harm
  - ◆ When expressed externally, anger is marked by aggression that can vary from mild indignation to violent rage
  - ◆ Anger can be released in positive or negative ways
    - ❭ Positive releases of anger include developing increased motivation to achieve, making changes, and developing confidence in oneself as well as in others' opinions
    - ❭ Negative releases of anger include cursing, using sarcasm, closing out further communication, and engaging in physical assault
  - ◆ Anger can be expressed internally or externally
    - ❭ Internal expression of anger may produce increased heart and respiratory rate, increased systolic and diastolic blood pressure, increased finger temperature, hyperactivity, tension, or hostility
    - ❭ External expression of anger may produce assertiveness, passivity, aggression, acting-out behavior, or rage
- Theories of anger have their roots in biology, psychology, and sociology
  - ◆ Biological theories of anger include the instinctual drive theory and the neurobiological theory
    - ❭ According to the *instinctual drive theory*, anger is an innate drive common to all animals
    - ❭ According to the *neurobiological theory*, neurotransmitters deep in the brain activate anger from other neural stimulation
  - ◆ Psychological theories of anger include the frustration-aggression theory and the behavioral theory
    - ❭ According to the *frustration-aggression theory*, a blocked or unattainable desire results in frustration, which causes aggressive behavior
    - ❭ According to the *behavioral theory*, aggression is learned early in life because it helps achieve goals
  - ◆ Sociocultural theories of anger include the social learning theory and the social environment theory
    - ❭ According to the *social learning theory*, social behavior developed through interacting with others teaches aggression
    - ❭ According to the *social environment theory*, expressions of anger are based on the social environment in which one lives; lack of personal territory increases aggressive behavior
- A person can successfully manage anger by responding directly to the problem, by using assertiveness training techniques, and by setting reasonable limits on behavior
  - ◆ Direct response refers to a person's conscious effort to reduce tension by engaging in physical activity (for example, taking a brisk walk alone or playing tennis or racquetball)

- ◆ Assertiveness training—a planned, conscious process to deal positively with anger—involves concrete steps
  - ❭ Analyze personal behavior
  - ❭ Record situations of assertive behavior
  - ❭ Observe how others react in similar situations
  - ❭ Identify alternative ways to handle situations
  - ❭ Try new alternatives
  - ❭ Get feedback on performance from others
- ◆ Setting limits helps prevent unreasonable expressions of anger that intrude on others
  - ❭ State acceptable boundaries of behavior
  - ❭ Express reasons for the anger
  - ❭ Develop alternative behaviors

❖ Grief

- ■ Grief is a powerful emotional reaction to a separation or loss, such as declining health, impending death, the death of a loved one, or the loss of a valuable personal object
- ■ Expressions of grief vary considerably, depending on one's personality, cultural background, and intensity of feeling toward the loss
- ■ Healthy grieving is time-limited, becoming less intense as time passes but taking 1 year or more to resolve fully
- ■ Grief can have physical, psychological, and social ramifications
  - ◆ Physical signs include insomnia; tight muscles, especially in the throat and chest; interrupted sleep; loss of appetite; and lethargy and generalized weakness
  - ◆ Psychological signs include preoccupation with or ambivalence toward the lost object, anger, fantasies that the object isn't lost, and guilt over inability to prevent the loss
  - ◆ Social signs include withdrawal from usual social activities and decreased work productivity
- ■ Healthy grieving consists of three stages: realization, disorganization, and resolution
  - ◆ In stage I (realization), shock, disbelief, and numbness initially overwhelm the person
    - ❭ The person becomes angry and resentful when others offer support
    - ❭ The person uses inner resources in an attempt to regain the lost object
    - ❭ The stage ends when the person gradually accepts the irreversibility of the loss
  - ◆ In stage II (disorganization), emotional pain from realization of the permanence of the loss creates disorganized behavior, loneliness, and a profound sense of helplessness
    - ❭ The person develops guilt over what could have been done to prevent the loss

▶ Crying, preoccupation with the lost object, despair, and loss of interest in social interactions are magnified
- ◆ In stage III (resolution), the bereaved person begins to think about life without the lost object
  - ▶ Emotional pain decreases, as evidenced by less crying and preoccupation with the loss
  - ▶ The person starts to develop a new lifestyle, focusing on new objects and new purposes for living
- ■ Dysfunctional grieving results from ambivalence toward the lost object, intolerance of the emotional pain of grieving, and social isolation; it requires professional intervention
  - ◆ Help the patient experience the emotions of grieving by exploring the importance of the lost object
  - ◆ Encourage the patient to recall memories of the lost object in order to identify and express the loss
  - ◆ Encourage the patient to express all feelings about the loss—even negative ones
  - ◆ Encourage the patient to develop independent relationships with others to talk about the loss in his or her own terms
  - ◆ Teach the patient how the grieving process functions
  - ◆ Help the patient develop goals for the future by focusing on individual strengths and abilities

❖ Coping

- ■ Coping is an individualized effort to understand and handle life's problems
- ■ Everyone develops resources to cope with stressors
  - ◆ The amount of coping effort required depends on how one evaluates the threat of the stressor in relation to one's inner coping abilities
  - ◆ Understanding a patient's appraisal of life's stressors and the coping resources developed is crucial to providing individualized nursing care
  - ◆ The coping resources that people use (first described by Mechanic, Lazarus, and Folkman) include individual skills and abilities, social support, economic resources, motivation, defensive techniques, personal health, and high self-esteem
  - ◆ Other coping resources include positive beliefs, problem-solving ability and social skills, and positive self-esteem
- ■ Coping mechanisms are the person's efforts to reduce stress and anxiety
  - ◆ A person may cope with mild anxiety through outbursts of temper, crying, vigorous exercise, fantasizing, or sleeping
  - ◆ More severe levels of anxiety, which become ego-threatening, require more extreme coping efforts such as the use of ego-centered defense mechanisms

▶ *Compensation* — emphasizing a perceived asset to make up for a perceived liability

▶ *Conversion* — the unconscious transfer of anxiety to a physical symptom that has no organic cause

▶ *Denial* — ignoring and refusing to recognize the reality of what's occurring in a person's life

▶ *Displacement* — transferring a feeling from an actual object or person to a more neutral one

▶ *Dissociation* — breaking off or separation of part of the personality from the rest of one's consciousness

▶ *Identification* — adopting the attributes of another person who is admired or perceived as an authority

▶ *Intellectualization* — using excessive cognition to ignore an unpleasant feeling

▶ *Projection* — attributing one's unacceptable thoughts or desires to another

▶ *Rationalization* — using excuses to justify undesirable behavior or thinking

▶ *Reaction formation* — demonstrating behavior that directly opposes one's true feelings

▶ *Regression* — reverting personality development to an earlier functional level

▶ *Repression* — removing undesirable thoughts or impulses from conscious awareness

▶ *Splitting* — perceiving people or situations that have a mix of positive and negative characteristics as being either completely positive or completely negative

▶ *Sublimation* — substituting an undesirable trait or impulse for one that's more socially acceptable

▶ *Substitution* — using an alternative source of satisfaction for one that isn't available

▶ *Suppression* — putting off awareness of disturbing feelings or situations (can be done on a conscious level)

◆ Destructive behavioral patterns dispel anxiety without resolving the cause

▶ *Neurotic behavior* — evidenced by distressing symptoms without socially unacceptable behavior and no reality testing impairment

▶ *Psychotic behavior* — characterized by a disintegrated personality, regressive behavior, disturbances in affect, and gross impairment of reality testing

❖ Transference and countertransference

■ *Transference* is an unconscious response in which the patient experiences feelings associated with a significant other earlier in life and transfers them to the therapist

◆ Transference is revealed during therapy and can help the patient in clarifying reality

◆ Two types of transference can intrude on a nurse-patient relationship

   ▶ In *hostile transference,* the patient directs hostility and rage internally by becoming discouraged with the therapeutic progress or externally by criticizing the therapist's capabilities

   ▶ In *dependent-reaction transference,* the patient becomes submissive and adoring and views the therapist as all-knowing and wise

■ *Countertransference* refers to projection of the therapist's feelings about a significant other to the patient during therapy

◆ Many patients provoke emotional reactions in the therapist

◆ The therapist may respond to these feelings through emotion or behavior that's inappropriate for and incongruent with the reality of the therapeutic situation

   ▶ Love reactions—involving oneself in the personal or social life of the patient

   ▶ Hostile reactions—showing anger or arguing with the patient

   ▶ Anxiety reactions—feeling guilty, uneasy, or nervous when interacting with the patient

◆ Countertransference can be therapeutically harmful and must be quickly addressed by the therapist

❖ Crisis and crisis intervention

■ *Crisis* refers to an imbalance in internal equilibrium that results from a stressor or threat to the self

◆ Crises develop from perceived or real losses, such as the death of a loved one, a job loss, or new challenges

◆ In 1964, Caplan identified four distinct phases of a crisis

   ▶ In phase I, the person identifies that a precipitating event has occurred

   ▶ In phase II, the ego perceives the degree of threat and tries to use previously successful coping methods

   ▶ In phase III, anxiety builds, thinking becomes disorganized, and the person develops a sense of helplessness

   ▶ In phase IV, the person organizes personal resources, tries new coping methods, or redefines the threat in a way that renders previously learned problem-solving techniques effective

◆ A person may experience one of three types of crisis

   ▶ Maturational crises are normally occurring events in life caused by the person's continual growth and development

   ▶ Situational crises are unexpected events (such as job loss or death of a loved one) that disrupt the biopsychosocial balance

   ▶ Social or adventitious crises are major cataclysmic disasters (such as an earthquake, a flood, or war) that cause a massive upheaval of social and personal order

■ *Crisis intervention* aims to restore the person to a precrisis level of functioning and order; its methods resemble the phases of the nursing process
  ◆ Assessment
    ▶ Identify the precipitating event
    ▶ Assess the patient's perception of the event
    ▶ Assess available coping skills and resources
    ▶ Assess the patient's level of anxiety as well as suicidal or homicidal potential
  ◆ Analysis and planning
    ▶ Organize assessment data
    ▶ Analyze the data
    ▶ Explore options to resolve the problem
    ▶ Decide on the steps needed to achieve the solution
  ◆ Implementation
    ▶ Change the patient's physical situation; provide emotional support and shelter
    ▶ Compare the nurse's perception of the problem with the patient's to clarify any misconceptions
    ▶ Secure economic and social resources by referring the patient to appropriate support groups
    ▶ Acknowledge the multiple feelings a patient has about the crisis to help the patient sort out and express his fears and expectations
    ▶ Help the patient develop and test possible solutions
  ◆ Evaluation
    ▶ Determine the effectiveness of implementations by observing behavioral outcomes and comparing them with goals
    ▶ Refer the patient for additional help if outcomes differ from those planned
■ Crisis intervention focuses on resolving the immediate crisis and requires the nurse's active involvement in numerous techniques
  ◆ *Abreaction (or catharsis)* — asking open-ended questions that will encourage the patient to express emotions about the crisis
  ◆ *Clarification* — helping the patient see the relationship between his problems and his feelings by encouraging him to express the cause (problem) and effect (his reaction)
  ◆ *Suggestion* — guiding a patient to accept a suggestion or idea that promotes self-confidence and optimism
  ◆ *Manipulation* — influencing a patient to benefit from the therapeutic intervention by using the patient's values
  ◆ *Reinforcement* — giving positive feedback when the patient makes healthy responses to the problem
  ◆ *Promoting self-esteem* — communicating confidently that the patient has the inner strength to find a solution to the problem

◆ *Support defenses* — assisting the patient to use positive defense mechanisms that promote self-esteem and ego strength rather than maladaptive defense mechanisms that deny or impair reality

◆ *Exploring solutions* — intently examining potential solutions to the problem with the patient

Review questions

1. The biochemical theory of anxiety specifically focuses on which of the following neurotransmitters?

○ **A.** GABA

○ **B.** Dopamine

○ **C.** Epinephrine

○ **D.** Serotonin

Correct answer: A GABA neurotransmitters have an inhibitory effect on anxiety.

2. Which of the following statements about anxiety is true?

○ **A.** Anxiety must be eliminated.

○ **B.** Moderate anxiety is helpful when taking examinations.

○ **C.** Mild anxiety can distort perceptions.

○ **D.** Mild anxiety enhances attention awareness.

Correct answer: D Mild anxiety enhances concentration and sharpens the ability to think and learn.

3. Which of the following statements could the nurse include in teaching a patient about anxiety?

○ **A.** "Anxiety is an abnormal state."

○ **B.** "Symptoms of anxiety should be hidden from others."

○ **C.** "Anxiety levels tend to be steady."

○ **D.** "Anxiety may be lowered by linking the manifested behavior with the feeling of anxiety."

Correct answer: D Anxiety is a universal part of human existence. Recognizing the manifested behavior caused by increased anxiety is one of the first steps in reducing anxiety.

4. Strategies for dealing with stress include:

   ❍ **A.** negative self-talk.

   ❍ **B.** daily use of gingko biloba.

   ❍ **C.** cutting back on exercising.

   ❍ **D.** daily use of kava-kava.

   Correct answer: D Kava-kava relieves anxiety and tension without affecting alertness. Gingko biloba is not known to have any effect on axiety. Cutting back on exercising and negative self-talk are not suggested strategies for dealing with stress.

5. Healthy grieving consists of which of the following three stages?

   ❍ **A.** Realization, disorganization, and resolution

   ❍ **B.** Disorganization, denial, and resolution

   ❍ **C.** Denial, anger, and bargaining

   ❍ **D.** Realization, anger, and resolution

   Correct answer: A The three stages of healthy grieving are realization of the loss, disorganization (helplessness), and resolution (beginning to cope).

Human development

❖ Overview
- ■ Human development proceeds in a cephalocaudal direction, from the simple to the complex
- ■ The developmental process is unique for each person, and what develops in the future depends on what has already happened
- ■ General theories of developmental behavior provide a foundation for examining the characteristics of the life cycle
- ■ Understanding the relative norms for important stages of development in the life cycle enables a nurse to assess whether a patient has made satisfactory progress within expected boundaries
- ■ Theoretical models focus on the psychoanalytic, psychosocial, and cognitive aspects of human development and provide concepts that guide the delivery of nursing care

❖ Psychoanalytic models of development
- ■ Freud, considered the father of psychoanalysis, described psychosexual development through adolescence; his model embraces four major tenets
  - ◆ All behavior holds some meaning about a person's personality
  - ◆ A person's personality consists of three parts
    - ❭ The *id*, the unconscious mind, operates instinctively and without control
    - ❭ The *ego*, the conscious mind, maintains contact with reality, examining all environmental and physiologic changes experienced by the person
    - ❭ The *superego* is the human conscience that directs and controls thoughts and feelings
  - ◆ To mature, a person must successfully traverse five stages of psychosexual development
    - ❭ During the *oral stage* (birth to 18 months), the child learns to handle anxiety by using the tongue and mouth
    - ❭ During the *anal stage* (18 months to age 3), the child learns to control muscles, especially those that control urination and defecation
    - ❭ During the *phallic (Oedipal) stage* (ages 3 to 6), the child learns sexual identity and becomes aware of the genital area

▶ During the *latency stage* (ages 6 to 12), the child experiences a relatively quiet phase when sexual development and energy are quiescent

▶ During the *genital stage* (age 12 to adulthood), sexual interest emerges as the person strives to develop satisfactory relationships with potential sex partners

◆ Unresolved conflicts at any stage of psychosexual development become fixated and remain part of the person's personality

■ In 1963, Erikson expanded Freud's work to encompass the life cycle and society's impact on development; the gradual growth of ego identity through the stages of development are based on social and cultural experiences culminating in a sense of humanity

◆ According to Erikson's model, psychosocial development is a series of conflicts that have favorable or unfavorable resolutions

◆ This development occurs in eight stages (with some degree of overlap)

▶ *Trust versus mistrust* (birth to age 1½): the child develops a sense of trust in or mistrust of others

● Consistent, affectionate care during this time produces a favorable resolution: trust in self and others

● Deficient, inconsistent care produces an unfavorable resolution: mistrust, withdrawal, and estrangement

▶ *Autonomy versus shame and doubt* (ages 1½ to 3): the child learns self-control or becomes self-conscious and full of doubt

● Praise, support, and encouragement in using newly acquired skills of independence and learning self-control favorably resolve this stage

● Shaming or insulting the child causes unnecessary dependence, compulsive self-restraint or compliance, or willfulness and defiance

▶ *Initiative versus guilt* (ages 3 to 6): the child initiates spontaneous activities or develops fear of wrongdoing

● Encouraging creative activities and giving clear explanations for events that occur in the child's life promote assertiveness and the sense of purpose necessary to move toward resolution of this stage

● Threatening punishment or labeling behavior as "bad" develops childhood guilt, fear of wrongdoing, lack of self-confidence, overcontrol and overrestriction of the child's activities

▶ *Industry versus inferiority* (ages 6 to 12): the child either develops the social and physical skills necessary to negotiate and compete in life or feels inadequate and inferior

● Recognizing the child's creative energy and sensitivity, and fostering activities that can be successfully completed build the confidence and competence to resolve this stage

- Unjust criticism or unreasonably high expectations create a sense of disappointment in one's own abilities as well as a feeling of inadequacy and inferiority
▶ *Identity versus role diffusion* (ages 12 to 20): the teenager either integrates childhood experiences into a personal identity or develops self-doubts about sexual or occupational roles
    - Helping the adolescent make decisions, encouraging active participation in home and school events, and assisting with future plans all help the teen actualize abilities and aid resolution of this stage
    - Not answering questions important to the teenager and imposing unilateral control over daily activities create doubt about sexual identity and personality confusion
▶ *Intimacy versus isolation* (ages 18 to 25): the person develops commitments to work and to other people or avoids close personal relationships and long-term lifestyle commitments
    - Teaching the young adult to achieve goals and foster personal relationships resolves this stage
    - Ridiculing romances or denigrating job selection causes the young adult to withdraw and avoid friendships, lifestyle commitments, and career
▶ *Generativity versus stagnation* (ages 21 to 45): the person either establishes a family and becomes creative and productive or lacks outside interests and becomes self-indulgent
    - Recognizing the person's responsibilities, providing emotional support, and praising achievements help resolve this stage
    - Failure at work, failure in intimate relationships, or lack of attachment to the community fosters self-indulgence, pseudointimacy, and detachment from society
▶ *Integrity versus despair* (age 45 to death): the person reviews life for meaning, fulfillment, and contributions made to the next generation or becomes dissatisfied with life, denies personal existence, and fears death
    - Exploring the positive aspects of one's life, such as contributions made and knowledge gained, successfully resolves this stage
    - Deciding that life has no meaning or purpose creates despair and hopelessness
- ◆ Unsuccessful passage through one stage influences passage through subsequent stages, creating the potential for psychosocial conflicts

❖ Cognitive and moral models of development
- ■ In 1963, Piaget postulated that human development evolves from cognition, learning, knowing, and comprehending
    - ◆ Biological changes, personal maturation, socialization, and life's experiences set the course for development

◆ Cognitive development is a continuous and orderly process, occurring in four stages

  ▶ *Sensorimotor* (birth to 1½ years): the child learns about himself and the immediate environment by exploring, discovering objects, and imitating others

  ▶ *Preoperational* (2 to 7 years): this stage is divided into two phases

   • *Preconceptional phase* (2 to 4 years): the child learns to think in terms of mental images and develops symbolic language and symbolic play

    • *Intuitive phase* (4 to 7 years): the child learns a rudimentary classification system by separating disparate objects and events and expands expressive language

  ▶ *Concrete operations* (ages 8 to 12): the child can systematically organize thoughts and facts about the environment, can apply rules to things that are seen and heard, and begins to engage in abstract thinking

  ▶ *Formal operations* (age 12 to adulthood): the person can think using conceptual, abstract operations and can hypothesize, test, and evaluate solutions to problems

■ Kohlberg emphasized cognitive development and social experience in the development of a personal morality, proposing six stages, or orientations, of moral development; two stages occur at each of three levels

  ◆ *Premoral level*

   ▶ *Obedience and punishment orientation:* the person obeys an authority figure and views misbehavior in terms of damage done

   ▶ *Instrumental relativist orientation:* the person defines "right" as that which is acceptable to and approved by the self

  ◆ *Conventional morality level*

   ▶ *Interpersonal concordance orientation:* the person maintains cordial human relations and the approval of others

   ▶ *Authority and duty orientation:* the person develops respect for authority and a duty to maintain the social order

  ◆ *Level of principled moral reasoning*

   ▶ *Social contract orientation:* the person accepts the morality of having democratically established laws

   ▶ *Universal ethics orientation:* the person understands the principles of human rights and personal conscience

❖ Interpersonal models of development

■ Sullivan theorized that interpersonal relations within a societal context influenced how one's life would develop

  ◆ Interpersonal growth is based on satisfying basic biological needs

  ◆ To form satisfactory relationships with others, one must complete six stages of development

   ▶ *Infancy stage* (birth to age 1½): the infant learns to rely on caregivers to meet desires and needs

▶ *Childhood stage* (ages 1½ to 6): the child learns to accept a delay in gratification of desires and needs

▶ *Juvenile stage* (ages 6 to 9): the child forms fulfilling relationships with peers

▶ *Preadolescence stage* (ages 9 to 12): the child successfully relates to same-sex companions

▶ *Early adolescence stage* (ages 12 to 14): the adolescent learns to be independent and to form congenial relationships with members of the opposite sex

▶ *Late adolescence stage* (ages 14 to 21): the person establishes a close, long-lasting relationship with someone of the opposite sex

■ In 1985, Stern postulated that children pass through four increasingly complex stages of self-relatedness during the first 2 years of life

◆ *Emergent self stage* (birth to 2 months): the infant begins to learn by making discriminating choices within the environment; developing awareness becomes the precursor for subsequent stages

◆ *Core self stage* (2 to 9 months): the infant begins to change the focus of interpersonal relationships away from himself and toward others, usually the caregivers

◆ *Subjective self stage* (9 to 18 months): the child commands attention in order to share experiences and develops the capacity to evaluate others' feelings toward him

◆ *Verbal self stage* (18 to 24 months): the child develops language skills that enhance interpersonal relationships

❖ **Life cycle characteristics**

■ Norms for growth and development usually are categorized according to widely accepted (albeit arbitrary) age ranges

■ Behavior patterns commonly overlap age ranges because each person's developmental process is unique

■ The nine age ranges, with prominent characteristics typically achieved at each range, are as follows:

◆ Infant (birth to age 1½)

▶ Rapidly developing motor skills highlight the early period, with physical development proceeding cephalocaudally, proximally to distally, and from general to specific movements

▶ Social-play skills emerge, giving the infant a strong sense of self and a distinct personality

▶ By the end of the period, the child can express affection and sympathy and likes to help with household chores

◆ Early child, or toddler (ages 1½ to 3)

▶ The child walks and explores the ever-growing world, becomes more coordinated, dances, rides a tricycle, and has a 900-word vocabulary

▶ Socially, the child begins this period by playing alone and using temper tantrums to control others; the child also imitates older children and fears strangers and desertion by caregivers

▶ By the end of the period, the child knows and identifies with his gender, plays with others, can tolerate brief separation from caregivers, and has participated in toilet training

◆ Middle child, or preschooler (ages 3 to 6)

▶ Physical growth slows and fine motor skills develop, characterized by the ability to skip, throw overhand, use scissors, and tie shoelaces

▶ Socially, the preschooler plays cooperatively, bathes and dresses independently, can be rude to others, and likes to fight

▶ A developing sense of conscience begins to control initiative; the child fears wrongdoing or parental disapproval

◆ Late child, or school-age child (ages 6 to 12)

▶ Physically, the child develops better motor skill control and more poise but still is awkward in trying new activities; height and weight increase; secondary sex characteristics begin to appear later in this period

▶ The child prefers associating with same-sex companions early in this period; competes but hates to lose; and can understand what society deems as unacceptable behavior but can't always choose between right and wrong without assistance

▶ Developing initiative and high self-esteem during this period helps the child acquire the skills needed to succeed in school

◆ Adolescent (ages 12 to 20)

▶ Physically, the teenager tires easily because the cardiovascular and respiratory systems develop more slowly than other body systems; sex characteristics blossom; dramatic physical growth produces clumsiness when it fails to adapt quickly enough to physical changes

▶ Adolescents enjoy partying and building independent relationships apart from the family

▶ Uncertainty about and inexperience in the working world make career selection difficult

◆ Young adult (ages 20 to 29)

▶ Today, young adulthood through age 30 is a kind of "provisional adulthood"; it's a period of psychosocial development in which the central task is to become differentiated from the family in which one grew up

▶ Both physical and higher order cognitive development have been completed

▶ Young adults may seek employment in the careers of their childhood dreams or experiment in the work force as the struggle for balance in integration of identity, role, and separation continues

◆ Adult (ages 30 to 45)

▶ At the peak of physical maturity when entering this period, the adult has minimal health concerns; energy and body function begin to diminish as the person gets older; proper nutrition, exercise, and rest help sustain well-being

▶ The adult assumes multiples roles, such as worker, lover, spouse, parent, and participant in the community

▶ The adult sorts out values and beliefs, discarding some of those learned earlier in favor of new ones; failure to achieve personal integration causes isolation later

◆ Middle adult (ages 45 to 65)

▶ Strength, physiologic reserve, and body systems continue to decline; dietary changes (for instance, less fat and more vitamins) become important; chronic diseases and sexual problems diminish self-esteem

▶ Social responsibilities widen to include parents, work associates, and neighbors; grown children leave home, creating an empty-nest syndrome

▶ Midlife crises occur, possibly spawning divorce, substance abuse, a new occupation, or changes in the way a person perceives his future role in life; the idealized self is replaced with a more realistic one; the person finds social value in life's accomplishments

◆ Late adult (age 65 to death)

▶ Physical functioning diminishes further; muscle tone and bone density decrease; vision and hearing losses result in reduced personal mobility; diminished sense of taste causes a loss of appetite, leading to nutritional imbalance; reductions in neurologic and sensory function impair reaction time

▶ The activity theory suggests that the level of activity in older adults may be influenced more by the individual's past lifestyle and social and economic forces than by the aging process itself.

▶ Retirement from employment changes the person's role identity, social activity, finances, and living habits; the deaths of friends and family reduce social contacts unless new ones are made

▶ The older adult evaluates the purpose of life and the contributions made to society; religion becomes more important as the older adult contemplates death more frequently; developing effective coping skills and a positive evaluation of one's contribution to society help create a strong sense of personal significance

Review questions

1. A 3-year-old boy has started preschool. On the third day, when his mother drops him off, he has a tantrum and refuses to walk by slumping down to the ground. According to Erikson, this behavior indicates which stage of psychosocial development?

◯ **A.** Initiative versus guilt

◯ **B.** Autonomy versus shame and doubt

◯ **C.** Industry versus inferiority

◯ **D.** Trust versus mistrust

Correct answer: B Autonomy versus shame and doubt is a typical conflict for a 3-year-old. The boy's tantrum results from his doubt and insecurity about participating in preschool activities.

2. The nurse is caring for an elderly gentleman in a skilled nursing center. He says to the nurse, "Why do you bother with me? I'm old and worthless." According to Erikson's theory, the patient is experiencing which of the following stages?

◯ **A.** Intimacy versus isolation

◯ **B.** Generativity versus stagnation

◯ **C.** Initiative versus guilt

◯ **D.** Integrity versus despair

Correct answer: D During the integrity-versus-despair stage of development, individuals over 45 may become dissatisfied with life. The patient expresses despair because he believes his life has no meaning.

3. A mother consults with the nurse about her 11-year-old daughter, who is spending all of her time with her girlfriend. The two girls have been friends through grade school and are more secretive lately about their activities. They also seem overly sarcastic about the boys in their class. The mother worries that her child may be engaging in inappropriate behavior. Using Sullivan's theory of development, the nurse's best response is to:

◯ **A.** inform the mother that the daughter is in the preadolescent stage of development.

◯ **B.** suggest that the daughter be tested psychologically.

◯ **C.** ask the mother more about her concerns because her daughter's secretiveness isn't normal.

◯ **D.** encourage the mother to invite her daughter, the girlfriend, and two boys to a picnic to observe the girls' interaction with the boys.

Correct answer: A According to Sullivan, preadolescence (ages 9 to 12) is a valuable developmental stage during which the child learns how to successfully relate to same-sex companions. The daughter's secretiveness may result from anxiety about sharing her conversations with adults.

4. Which of the following statements is a tenet of Freud's psychoanalytic theory?

   ○ **A.** All behavior holds some meaning about a person's personality.

   ○ **B.** Psychosocial development is a series of conflicts that have favorable or unfavorable resolutions.

   ○ **C.** Human development evolves from cognition, learning, knowing, and comprehension.

   ○ **D.** Children pass through four increasingly complex stages of self-relatedness during the first 2 years of life.

Correct answer: A Options B, C, and D are theories associated with Erikson, Piaget, and Stern, respectively.

5. The nurse is orienting a recently admitted patient to the psychiatric unit. She discusses the rules of the unit with the patient so that a social milieu can be maintained for the benefit of all patients. The client says, "I don't have to obey the rules. My psychiatrist said I am more sophisticated than other patients and the rules don't apply to me." The nurse's response to the patient should focus on which of the following stages of Kolhberg's theory of moral development?

   ○ **A.** Authority and duty orientation

   ○ **B.** Obedience and punishment orientation

   ○ **C.** Universal ethics orientation

   ○ **D.** Intrapersonal concordance orientation

Correct answer: A During the stage of authority and duty orientation, individuals develop respect for authority and a duty to maintain social order. The nurse's reply to the patient should establish social order, which is a part of a therapeutic milieu.

CHAPTER 4

Settings, roles, and scope of practice

❖ Overview

- Modern psychiatric nursing practice emerged in 1946 with the creation of the National Institute of Mental Health (NIMH) and the authorization of psychiatric nursing education grants by the federal government
- Graduate programs in psychiatric and mental health nursing proliferated throughout American universities
- As the educational level of psychiatric nurses increased, roles expanded for advanced practice nurses and opportunities for nurses to practice in different and more varied settings increased
- Contemporary psychiatric and mental health nursing practice in its current varied roles became official when the NIMH recognized psychiatric nursing as a legitimate mental health discipline

❖ Practice settings

- Psychiatric and mental health nurses work in a wide range of practice settings
- Hospitals provide a patient-restrictive setting in which the patient receives intense treatment and constant monitoring
- Transitional facilities offer partial hospitalization and intense therapy for a patient who is psychiatrically stable enough to forgo traditional hospitalization
- Outpatient clinics provide various assessment and treatment services and typically involve a brief stay (a few hours or a day)
- Community mental health centers provide individual, family, and group therapy; aftercare consultation and education; and treatment and rehabilitation for addiction disorders
- The patient's home serves as the practice setting for community mental health nurses, who visit periodically to evaluate the patient's adaptation to community life and to conduct patient teaching
- Health maintenance organizations (HMOs) serve as case managers to support the patient's highest level of functioning

❖ **Functional roles and role components**
- Psychiatric and mental health nurses provide direct care (carrying out nursing tasks) and indirect care (supervising others, assigning staff, handling staff conflicts and stressors)
- In 1994, the American Nurses Association's (ANA's) Division on Psychiatric and Mental Health Nursing Practice issued a statement on standards of psychiatric and mental health clinical nursing practice and nursing activities (see *Psychiatric nursing activities*)
- Psychiatric and mental health nurses assume various roles when providing care
  ◆ Provider of direct or indirect nursing care
  ◆ Coordinator of care
  ◆ Supervisor
  ◆ Nursing administrator
  ◆ Consultant and collaborator
  ◆ Staff and patient educator
  ◆ Patient advocate
  ◆ Researcher
  ◆ Case manager
  ◆ Advanced practitioners (such as clinical specialist or nurse practitioner)
- Psychiatric and mental health nurses provide a variety of major services known as role components, seven of which are universal to all practice settings
  ◆ Planning and implementing care through a therapeutic relationship
  ◆ Managing the socioenvironment
  ◆ Administering and monitoring drugs
  ◆ Assisting patients with activities of daily living
  ◆ Educating patients and families
  ◆ Facilitating family and group interaction
  ◆ Working with an interdisciplinary team

❖ **Scope of practice**
- Psychiatric and mental health nursing practice involves working with a multidisciplinary mental health team
  ◆ A nurse can be a member of three classes of teams
    ▶ *Unidisciplinary* team members are from the same discipline
    ▶ *Multidisciplinary* team members are from different disciplines, each providing specific patient services
    ▶ *Interdisciplinary* team members are from different disciplines, formally organized to provide coordinated care based on the unique contribution of each team member
  ◆ Nurses are commonly designated the team leader because they're always present in the patient environment
  ◆ Mental health teams include several specialists
    ▶ Psychiatrist, who specializes in the treatment of mental illnesses

---

Psychiatric nursing activities

Psychiatric and mental health nurses engage in various activities to promote the patient's well-being. Primary activities recognized by the American Nurses Association include:

- emphasizing health promotion and health maintenance
- performing intake screening and evaluation
- functioning in the case manager role
- providing a therapeutic milieu

- monitoring and promoting self-care activities
- administering and monitoring psychobiological interventions
- providing health teaching, crisis care, and psychiatric rehabilitation.

Adapted from American Nurses Association, *Scope and Standards of Psychiatric-Mental Health Nursing Practice*. Washington, D.C., 2000, with permission of the publisher.

▶ Advanced practice nurse, who works cooperatively with the doctor to diagnose and treat common mental health problems
▶ Psychiatric nurse, who specializes in managing the patient environment and giving 24-hour care
▶ Clinical psychologist, who specializes in diagnostic testing of mental processes
▶ Psychiatric social worker, who specializes in family and social evaluation of the causes of patient illnesses
▶ Psychiatric technician, who assists nurses in giving care and meeting the patient's basic needs
▶ Dietitian, who specializes in developing and providing a nourishing diet for the patient
▶ Expressive therapist (or creative arts therapist), who specializes in the use of art, music, movement, or other therapies that enable the client to identify and work on resolving complex issues
▶ Occupational therapist, who specializes in assessing the patient's ability to perform useful tasks that contribute to patient resocialization
▶ Recreational therapist, who specializes in assessing the patient's ability to engage in leisure activities (such as hobbies and sports) that contribute to the patient's resocialization
▶ Spiritual advisor, who specializes in meeting the patient's spiritual needs
▶ Patient, who is the focus of the care plan and who participates in decisions about care if able
◆ Barriers to effective team functioning can occur if individual team members' roles and functions aren't agreed on by the whole team; Benfar has described three obstacles to effective team functioning
  ▶ Poor identification of roles and functions
  ▶ Inability to resolve role overlaps
  ▶ Intrateam communication problems

◆ For a team to work therapeutically, each member must know three things
- ▶ The goals that have been established
- ▶ The specific therapeutic activities that will be provided
- ▶ The effects of therapeutic activities on the patient's goals

◆ Team members should know the principles of collaborative (interdisciplinary) practice
- ▶ All team members focus on and contribute to the patient outcomes
- ▶ The patient participates in team meetings if able
- ▶ Specific functions of each discipline are unique and yet overlap with other disciplines

■ A major role of the psychiatric and mental health nurse is to provide leadership for a group

◆ The group may be a unit nursing staff, a mental health team, a quality assurance committee, or a community group

◆ There are several ways an effective leader can influence group activities to achieve goals
- ▶ Communicating group goals clearly
- ▶ Motivating group participants to excel
- ▶ Initiating new ideas about how to reach group goals
- ▶ Helping group members express feelings and concerns
- ▶ Integrating the group's achievements into a greater organizational structure

◆ Primary leadership roles involve several elements
- ▶ *Communication* — transmitting information between two or more people and between organizational levels
- ▶ *Delegation* — giving responsibility to others for completing assignments
- ▶ *Education* — teaching others new skills and knowledge
- ▶ *Innovation* — being a change agent by taking risks to try new techniques and procedures to achieve goals
- ▶ *Control* — monitoring outcomes to ensure that goals are being met

◆ A leader typically displays one of three styles of leadership
- ▶ *Authoritarian style* — a rigidly structured, rule-oriented approach with the focus on the leader, who clearly is in charge
- ▶ *Democratic style* — collaborative direction with group members; shared decision making and member-centered focus
- ▶ *Laissez-faire style* — little or no direction; leaves group members to their own resources; unsure of goals

◆ Effective leadership is more likely under the following conditions
- ▶ Group goals are clearly defined
- ▶ Group members agree on goals
- ▶ Goals are measurable
- ▶ Group goals coincide with personal and organizational goals
- ▶ Group expectations are clearly known

▶ Expectations are organizationally compatible
▶ Group expectations can be met

■ Performance improvement—the scope of nursing practice encompassing the quality of patient care compared with accepted industry standards—is known as quality or performance improvement (formerly quality assurance)

◆ Quality measurement activities can enhance patient health outcomes in both acute-care and outpatient settings

◆ Performance improvement is a natural process for the nurse to embrace because it encompasses principles that nurses are accustomed to applying in everyday practice: the nursing process steps of assessing, planning, implementing, and reevaluating

◆ The goal of performance improvement is to improve the quality of patient care and patient health outcomes using a planned, systems-oriented approach that focuses on organizational processes, not on individual performance

▶ A systematic approach includes the following components
  • Process design (can include designing a new service or evaluating a current clinical process or other internal process)
  • Performance measurement (includes identifying the processes to be measured and collecting relevant data)
    – Processes to be considered include but aren't limited to high cost, high volume, and problem-prone issues
    – According to the Joint Commission on Accreditation of Healthcare Organizations (JCAHO) standards, measurement of important functions of health care should be ongoing
    – Sources of data collection for performance measurement can include patient surveys, risk management activities, quality control activities, infection control statistics, employee or organizational feedback, and committee activities
  • Performance assessment (converts data into information; uses preestablished standards of care, performance expectations, design specifications, and other relevant criteria as a reference point for comparison of data and performance)
    – Comparisons can be based on internal, historical databases; external databases; or best practices (benchmarking)
    – Performance assessment includes identification of reasons for process variation (common cause versus special cause variation) as well as the use of statistical control tools (run charts, control charts) to understand variation
    – Performance assessment identifies the need for further assessment or study based on patterns and trends, the variability of performance levels outside the expected range, or a "sentinel event"
  • Performance improvement (stematic approach taken to improve an existing process)

— Priorities for process improvements must be established by the leaders of the organization

— The organization must determine the dimensions of performance to be improved as identified by JCAHO: efficacy, appropriateness, availability, timeliness, effectiveness, continuity, safety, efficiency, respect, and caring

— Various process improvement models and methods can be used, depending on the organization's preference (JCAHO 10-Step Process; PDSA [Plan, Do, Study, Act] Cycle; FOCUS [Find a process to improve, Organize a team that knows the process, Clarify current knowledge, Understand variation, Select a potential process improvement]; FADE [Focus, Analyze, Develop, Execute]; IMPROVE [Identify and define the problem, Measure the impact on customers, Prioritize possible causes, Research and analyze root causes, Outline alternative solutions, Validate that solutions will work, Execute solutions and standardize])

❭ Psychiatric and mental health nurses are held accountable and responsible for participating in quality improvement activities, thus ensuring improved patient health outcomes and patient satisfaction

- Identifying a potential opportunity for improvement
- Testing a strategy for change
- Assessing data to determine whether an improvement has occurred
- Implementing the improvement systemwide

❭ In response to current health care financing issues and the Health Care and Political Agenda for Change, improving health care and patient outcomes is motivated by numerous factors

- Consumers' perceptions of quality
- Managed care companies evaluating such features as accessibility and availability, quality of services rendered, and member satisfaction
- Federal and state requirements regarding specific quality measurements, member satisfaction surveys, complaint logs, and outcome reviews
- Peer review organizations to review HMO inpatient and ambulatory care

■ The scope of practice for a psychiatric and mental health nurse also includes psychiatric evaluation of patients who present themselves to the health care system

◆ Knowledge of human behavior, psychopathology, and psychotherapy equips the psychiatric and mental health nurse to perform the initial evaluation and then arrange for care by other members of the mental health team

◆ The psychiatric evaluation determines a patient's danger to himself or others, ability to provide self-care, and degree of reality impairment

◆ It precisely describes the patient's emotional and intellectual functioning at a specific time

◆ The evaluation is conducted during a private interview; the nurse listens attentively and observes the patient closely

◆ A psychiatric evaluation has three components

  ▶ Identifying the presenting problem

   • Obtain the patient's description of the presenting problem

   • Determine the problem's onset

   • Obtain the patient's perception of the problem

   • Determine the patient's perception of what caused the problem

  ▶ Taking a history

   • Medical

   • Family

   • Social

   • Psychiatric

   • Personal

  ▶ Performing a mental status examination

   • Note the patient's appearance, reaction to the interview, and outward behavior

   • Note level of consciousness, short- and long-term memory recall, orientation, judgment, insight, and intellectual functioning

   • Observe speech characteristics, thought patterns, and manner of communication

   • Observe affect for intensity and appropriateness

   • Note mood, looking especially for suicidal or homicidal ideation

   • Assess the patient's insight and understanding of the problem

◆ Data are then organized and analyzed

◆ Medical and nursing diagnoses are made

◆ Development of a treatment plan completes the evaluation process

❖ Advanced practice nursing

■ Advanced practice registered nursing is characterized by autonomous practice and the exercise of sophisticated levels of independent judgment

■ Nurses in advanced practice diagnose health problems, initiate care plans, and prescribe treatment plans

■ A nurse in advanced practice has graduate-level education in a specific area of nursing, had supervised practice during graduate education, and possesses continual clinical experience

■ The scope of advanced practice nursing is governed by federal and state laws and regulations, a professional code of ethics, professional practice standards, and the nurse's own competence as determined by education, experience, knowledge, and ability

  ◆ Advanced practice roles

▶ Clinical nurse specialist (an expert in a specific clinical area who acts as a patient advocate, provides direct patient care, teaches patients and families, conducts research, and acts as a consultant)

▶ Nurse-anesthetist (a certified registered nurse anesthetist who provides anesthesia and anesthesia-related care, including preanesthetic preparation and anesthesia induction, maintenance, and emergence)

▶ Nurse-midwife (possesses the education, clinical judgment, and skills to manage the care of pregnant women and newborns)

▶ Nurse practitioner (an educated and knowledgeable health care provider who can exercise critical judgment in assessing, diagnosing, and prescribing treatment in the clinical management of acute and chronic health problems)

◆ Advanced practice settings
  ▶ Medical centers
  ▶ Communities
  ▶ Schools
  ▶ Ambulatory settings
  ▶ Work sites
  ▶ Independent offices

◆ Advanced practice education
  ▶ Graduate-level education in theory and experience
  ▶ Supervised graduate-level practice

◆ Certification for advanced practice
  ▶ Provides national recognition of professional competence
  ▶ Requires graduation from an approved educational program that offers didactic and clinical experience in the specialty

◆ Advanced practice regulation
  ▶ Practice is regulated by appropriate state and federal laws and regulations
  ▶ State nurse practice acts provide the necessary legal umbrella for advanced practice nursing

◆ Advanced practice ethics
  ▶ Ethical decisions and ethical actions are the cornerstone of advanced practice nursing
  ▶ Advanced practice nurses respect the rights of patients to determine the level of care they receive, to privacy and confidentiality, to truthful disclosure of all treatment options and potential outcomes, and to dignity
  ▶ Nurses in advanced practice help patients make decisions, establish an ethical environment, and promote professional ethics

■ Standards of advanced practice
  ◆ The ANA has cooperated with specialty nursing organizations to develop standards of nursing practice
  ◆ Standards for advanced practice registered nursing have been promulgated by the ANA

◆ Specialty nursing organization standards give a detailed standard of practice for respective specialty practice

◆ Standards define the professional responsibilities of the advanced practice nurse to the public and the patient

◆ Standards of advanced practice consist of standards of care and standards of professional performance

▶ Standards of care

- *Assessment* — collection of comprehensive health data on a patient
- *Diagnosis* — analysis of the assessment data to establish a diagnosis
- *Outcome identification* — identifying the expected outcomes of treatment based on risks, benefits, and costs
- *Planning* — development of a comprehensive patient care plan
- *Implementation* — prescribing and ordering treatment interventions for the care plan
- *Case management* — providing coordinated, comprehensive care services consistent with quality and cost-effectiveness
- *Consultation* — providing advice and influence to improve the patient care plan
- *Health promotion and maintenance* — teaching strategies to promote and maintain an optimum level of wellness and prevent illness and injury
- *Prescriptive authority* — prescribing and authorizing drugs and treatments according to law to treat illness and restore health function
- *Referral* — identifying the need for care by other expert practitioners
- *Evaluation* — evaluating patient progress in achieving planned outcomes

▶ Standards of professional performance

- *Quality of care* — developing criteria for measuring the effectiveness of advanced practice
- *Performance appraisal* — evaluating self and peers and evaluating practice in relation to established standards and norms for competent clinical care
- *Education* — acquiring new skills and maintaining current knowledge in the specialty area
- *Leadership* — serving as a role model and leader for peers, colleagues, and others
- *Ethics* — using ethical principles in dealing with patients and professional peers
- *Interdisciplinary process* — building a respectful interdisciplinary process with other health care team members
- *Research* — using research to examine theories of care and develop new approaches to practice

Review questions

1. The nurse-supervisor calls a staff meeting to address a problematic situation on the unit. The democratic leadership style of the nurse is evident by which of the following actions?

○ **A.** She hands out a written report addressing the acceptable solutions.

○ **B.** She assembles work groups to discuss and propose ideas about the issue.

○ **C.** She addresses the concern by using the established method of problem solving.

○ **D.** She states that management will address the circumstances that created the problem.

Correct answer: B A democratic style of leadership is demonstrated by a leader who requests member input and focuses on shared decision making.

2. A nurse serves on a quality and performance improvement team in the hospital where she's employed. Which of the following types of work would the nurse perform?

○ **A.** Collecting data on the existing conditions related to the issue of concern

○ **B.** Retrieving old records to change the information that they contain

○ **C.** Directing the staff to try a change and report findings to the team

○ **D.** Writing a letter to the nursing administrator documenting patient complaints

Correct answer: A A quality performance team collects data on a project to determine the extent of compliance with agency goals and mission statement or accepted industry standards.

3. Two major responsibilities of the advanced practice registered nurse are to coordinate the services necessary for maintaining the patient's health and to provide high-quality, cost-effective services. These responsibilities fall under which standard of care?

○ **A.** Interdisciplinary process

○ **B.** Outcome identification

○ **C.** Prescriptive authority

○ **D.** Case management

Correct answer: D Case management consists of providing coordinated, comprehensive care services consistent with quality and cost-effectiveness. Outcome identification refers to the nurse identifying the expected outcomes of treatment based on risks, benefits, and costs. Prescriptive authority involves prescribing drugs and treatments to treat illness and restore the patient's health. The interdisciplinary process is a standard of professional performance, not a standard of care.

4. An advanced practice nurse works in a community mental health clinic serving a population that needs drug and alcohol services. The nurse's responsibilities in this practice setting include which of the following?

○ **A.** Intensive rehabilitative follow-up

○ **B.** Evaluation of somatic complaints

○ **C.** Assessment, treatment, and referral

○ **D.** Management of psychosocial environment

Correct answer: C Community health centers provide individual, family, and group therapy, aftercare consultation and education, and treatment and rehabilitation for addiction disorders. A major role of the nurse in a community mental health clinic is to assess, diagnose, and treat or refer patients to appropriate health care resources.

5. The nurse reviews a patient's progress in achieving his planned outcomes. The nurse is demonstrating which of the following ANA standards of psychiatric and mental health clinical nursing care?

○ **A.** Implementation

○ **B.** Interdisciplinary process

○ **C.** Quality of care

○ **D.** Evaluation

Correct answer: D Evaluation is the process of determining the patient's progress in achieving planned outcomes. Implementation is the prescribing and ordering of treatment interventions for the patient's care plan. Interdisciplinary process and quality of care are standards of professional performance, not standards of care.

Theoretical models of behavior

❖ **Overview**
- Human behavior is best understood within a conceptual framework
- A strong theoretical grounding provides the practitioner with an understanding of behavioral psychopathology and promotes thoughtful and logical practice
- Nine models and two theories of human behavior are widely used; because human behavior isn't fully understood, no model or theory is considered right or wrong, better or worse than any other model or theory
- The practitioner's theoretical perspective will determine the conceptual model selected in developing a care plan
- Psychiatric and mental health nurses commonly use an eclectic approach, drawing on several theoretical models of behavior, to fashion practical and effective care plans

❖ **Psychoanalytic model**
- Freud is considered the father of psychoanalytic theory
- His theory states that deviations in human behavior result from unsuccessful task accomplishment during earlier developmental stages
- Freud's psychoanalytic theory of behavior is built on five assumptions
  - ◆ The personality consists of three structures: id, ego, and superego
    - ▶ The *id* is present at birth
      - The id houses a person's needs, drives, and wishes
      - Because the id always seeks immediate reduction from tension, it operates on the pleasure principle
      - The id isn't oriented to reality
    - ▶ The *ego* begins to form between ages 4 and 5 months
      - The ego develops because the id must negotiate with external reality to meet its needs
      - The ego mediates between the id and external reality
      - The ego operates in reality and can solve problems
      - To protect itself from being overwhelmed by anxiety, the ego uses defense mechanisms such as repression
    - ▶ The *superego* begins to develop at age 3
      - The superego is an outgrowth of the ego
      - It houses the conscience, one's inner sense of right and wrong

- Like the id, the superego isn't reality oriented; it's concerned with the ideal and is rather rigid and moralistic in its application of what's right or wrong

◆ Development occurs in five stages, during which the child must master specific psychosexual conflicts to become a healthy, functioning adult; the names of the stages reflect the body area most associated with the child's source of gratification

▶ The *oral stage* occurs between birth and age 18 months
  - The child's needs are satisfied by oral gratification: feeding, exploring objects by placing them in the mouth, or exploring by using the lips
  - If needs are met, the child gains a feeling of trust and well-being
  - If needs aren't met satisfactorily, the child becomes an adult who is afraid and ill at ease

▶ The *anal stage* occurs between ages 18 months and 3 years
  - The child develops an awareness of fullness in the rectum
  - The child takes pleasure in retaining or eliminating feces
  - If this stage is negotiated effectively, the child becomes an adult who can delay gratification to attain future goals
  - If this stage is inadequately negotiated, the child becomes an adult who is either excessively rigid and conservative or messy and destructive

▶ The *phallic (Oedipal) stage* occurs between ages 3 and 6
  - The child takes pleasure in exploring and manipulating genitalia
  - The child is attracted to the opposite-sex parent but realizes that he can't sexually relate with this parent; the dilemma is resolved by identifying with the same-sex parent
  - During this stage, the superego develops and the conscience is formed
  - If needs are adequately met during this stage, the child develops a sex-appropriate identity and well-differentiated superego
  - If needs are inadequately met during this stage, the child becomes an adult whose sexual identity is confused and has problems relating to authority figures

▶ The *latency stage* occurs between ages 6 and 12
  - The child has learned to express inner drives and urges in socially acceptable ways; sexual tension is sublimated into age-appropriate activities
  - If this stage is successfully negotiated, the child becomes an adult who can deal with various life situations
  - If this stage isn't successfully negotiated, the child becomes an adult who has difficulty developing social skills and who feels inferior to others

▶ The *genital stage* occurs between ages 13 and 20

● Corresponding with genital maturation is a reawakening of the sex drive

● The child expends energy establishing psychological independence from his parents and family

● If this stage is completed successfully, an adult emerges whose personality structure is integrated, allowing the development of love and work relationships

● Unsuccessful completion of this stage results in an adult whose ability to establish intimacy and a strong personal identity is greatly compromised

◆ Mental or psychological activity occurs on three levels

▶ The *conscious level* houses part of the ego

● The conscious mind is much smaller than the unconscious mind

● The conscious mind is reality-based

● Any mental information readily available to the individual is located in the conscious

▶ The *subconscious level* houses part of the ego

● The subconscious acts as a filtering device between the external environment and the ego and between the unconscious and the ego

● Information stored in the subconscious can be called into conscious awareness

▶ The *unconscious level* houses the id and part of the superego

● Comparatively, the unconscious mind is much larger than the conscious mind

● The unconscious isn't reality-based

● Information housed in the unconscious affects behavior; the information is unavailable to the conscious mind

◆ Behavior is motivated by anxiety, the cornerstone of psychopathology

▶ Anxiety arises when unresolved conflicts are stimulated

● To protect itself against overwhelming anxiety, the ego enacts defense mechanisms

● Deviant behavioral symptoms result from these defense mechanisms

▶ Severe anxiety may produce behavioral regression to an earlier developmental level

● If regression occurs, the individual uses more primitive defense mechanisms

● This compromises the individual's ability to function at an age-appropriate level

◆ Behavior is always meaningful and often unconsciously motivated

■ The psychoanalytic model holds numerous implications for the nurse

◆ Understanding the psychosexual stages of childhood provides a framework for understanding behaviors observed in adult patients

◆ Effective parenting can be promoted by teaching parents about the child's needs during each psychosexual stage

◆ Successfully identifying manifestations of anxiety and the defense mechanisms used to control anxiety provides a premise for planning nursing care

◆ Defense mechanisms protect a patient from overwhelming anxiety; the nurse shouldn't deliberately interfere with them

◆ All behavior is meaningful, commonly representing the unconscious needs and wishes of patients who don't always know why they behave as they do

❖ Interpersonal models

■ Sullivan and Peplau are prominent interpersonal theorists

■ Sullivan believed that human development results from interpersonal relationships and that behavior is motivated by the avoidance of anxiety and the attainment of satisfaction

◆ He described three modes by which people relate to the external world

▶ The *prototaxic mode,* the most primitive mode, is used mainly by infants, who don't yet view themselves as differentiated individuals

▶ The *parataxic mode* is commonly used by children and juveniles, who view themselves as differentiated from the world but don't clearly understand how they and the rest of the world fit together

▶ The *syntaxic mode,* the highest mode of relating, is used by older children and adults, who can understand complex situations and use consensual validation

◆ Sullivan believed that the *self system* (akin to the ego in Freud's psychoanalytic model) is designed to protect one against anxiety and to allow one to obtain satisfaction; the self system has three components

▶ The "good me" makes approved behaviors part of the self; self-identification is positive

▶ The "bad me" identifies disapproved behaviors that, if carried out, would be viewed as negative by the self

▶ The "not me" denies the existence of behaviors that, if identified with the self, would arouse intense anxiety

◆ Sullivan outlined six stages of growth and development; within each stage, the person possesses the tools for completing the developmental tasks central to any given stage (see "Interpersonal models of development," chapter 3, page 21)

◆ Sullivan's interpersonal model holds numerous implications for the nurse

▶ The nurse can strengthen the "good me" by assisting the patient to develop positive behaviors

▶ Teaching patients how to use consensual validation assists them to function in the syntaxic mode

▶ If a patient's world view is fragmented (parataxic mode), a corrective relationship with the nurse will promote the patient's ability to relate to the world on an integrated (syntaxic mode) level

▶ Exploration of a behavior isn't as important as exploration of the anxiety associated with that behavior

▶ The nurse can design corrective experiences aimed at reversing developmental deficiencies

■ Peplau drew on Sullivan's theory to propose an interpersonal nursing theory that advanced the practice of psychiatric nursing by defining it as an interpersonal process

◆ She proposed that nurses must promote the nurse-patient relationship to build trust and foster healthy behavior

◆ She demonstrated how nurses could use psychodynamic concepts and counseling techniques with patients

◆ Peplau maintained that the therapeutic use of self promotes healing

◆ Through examination of the nurse-patient relationship, both nurse and patient benefit from the therapeutic relationship

▶ The therapeutic relationship is directed toward meeting the patient's needs and is thus patient focused

▶ All nurses must examine their responses to patients, but they should never be the focus of the therapeutic relationship

▶ Consistency in the nurse-patient relationship fosters the development of trust

▶ Nurses are accountable to patients for the quality of their work during the nurse-patient therapeutic relationship

▶ The nurse-patient relationship moves through four distinct phases

• In the *orientation phase,* the nurse establishes the parameters of the relationship

• In the *identification phase,* the patient describes the problem

• In the *exploitation phase,* the nurse and the patient examine the problem within the context of the therapeutic relationship

• In the *resolution phase,* the nurse and the patient summarize progress made in resolving the problem and formally terminate the relationship

◆ Believing anxiety to be an important motivator of behavior, Peplau classified anxiety into four levels

▶ *Mild anxiety* is characterized by heightened perception, increased alertness and awareness, and enhanced learning; it may also produce restlessness or irritability

▶ *Moderate anxiety* is characterized by a narrowed perceptual field and decreased alertness and concentration; physical symptoms include increased heart and respiratory rate, muscle tension, gastric discomfort, and voice tremors

▶ *Severe anxiety* is characterized by a greatly reduced perceptual field, extremely limited attention span, inability to learn, and markedly impaired problem-solving ability; symptoms include headache, nausea, trembling, insomnia, hyperventilation, urinary frequency, and diarrhea

> *Panic anxiety* is characterized by a perceptual field that demonstrates total inability to focus, loss of ability to see environmental details, concentrate, comprehend, or learn; symptoms may include dilated pupils, labored breathing, diaphoresis, pallor, immobility or hyperactivity, incoherence, and inability to verbalize

◆ Peplau's interpersonal model has these implications

> The therapeutic relationship serves as a corrective experience that the patient can use as a building block in developing other successful relationships

> The nurse uses empathy to access the patient's feelings

> The nurse uses the self as a therapeutic tool to enhance the patient's growth; a by-product is the nurse's personal growth

> Nursing is an interpersonal process in which the nurse and the patient affect and are affected by each other

> Anxiety is interpersonally communicated

> Anxiety affects the patient's ability to perceive a situation objectively and to generate alternatives

❖ Social model

■ Caplan and Szasz, the theorists of this model, postulate that the entire sociocultural environment influences mental health

■ The social model embraces four fundamental principles

◆ Deviant human behavior is defined by the culture in which a person lives

> Szasz described the "myth" of mental illness, whereby a society labels someone considered undesirable as mentally ill

> This label, in effect, helps control undesirables by hospitalizing them

> Undesirable or abnormal behavior in one society may be considered normal in another society

◆ People can control whether they desire to conform to societal expectations

◆ Physical pathology defines illness and influences behavior but doesn't cause deviant behavior

◆ Crises precipitate deviant behavior because a person is vulnerable to sociocultural stress

■ Caplan proposed that social conditions and interactions (family strife, poverty, inadequate education) dispose people to mental illness

■ He applied primary, secondary, and tertiary health prevention principles to mental health

◆ Primary prevention involves avoiding disease

◆ Secondary prevention involves shortening a disease episode

◆ Tertiary prevention involves controlling the adverse impact of disease

- Nursing implications of the social model
  - ◆ The nurse collaborates with the patient to change behavior
  - ◆ The patient may accept or reject the plan to solve the problem
  - ◆ Therapeutic interventions are influenced by the sociocultural environment
  - ◆ The nurse has a moral obligation to provide mental health services that address all health prevention levels
  - ◆ The therapeutic approach involves using the entire social context of the patient's life
  - ◆ Increased community involvement by the nurse enhances understanding of the patient's environment

❖ Existential model
- This theory centers on a person's present experiences rather than on past ones
- Frankl, Perls, and May exerted much influence on existential theory
- The existential model is based on four principles
  - ◆ Alienation from the self causes deviant behavior
  - ◆ The self imposes behavioral restrictions that cause the alienation
  - ◆ Each person can make free choices about which behaviors to display
  - ◆ People submit to others' demands rather than be themselves
- Existential theory relies heavily on the assumption that people can make free choices from life's table of offerings
- Nursing implications of the existential model
  - ◆ The patient has free choice of what's available in life
  - ◆ The nurse works to help the patient return from a state of self-alienation to a state of full life
  - ◆ The nurse and the patient are equals in humanity as they deal with the patient's problem
  - ◆ Human caring and a warm attitude help encourage the patient to test different behaviors

❖ Nursing model
- Several prominent theorists—including Rogers, Orem, Sister Roy, and Peplau—introduced models for nursing care that emphasized the person as a biopsychosocial being
- This holistic approach draws on general systems, developmental, and interactive theories to promote nursing care characterized by collaboration between the patient and the nurse
- The nursing model focuses on caring (in contrast to other models, which focus on curing)
- A central premise of the nursing model is that people live within a biopsychosocial framework that decides their health state

■ The nurse assesses a patient's physical and emotional behavior, interprets the patient's needs to others caring for the patient, and changes the biopsychosocial framework to meet the patient's needs

■ The nursing process is based on the holistic perspective of the nursing model

◆ Assessment (data collection) includes developing a health history of the patient's physical or psychological problem

◆ Analyzing the data and formulating the nursing diagnoses require the nurse to consider all the physical, social, and emotional stressors that contributed to the deviant behavior

◆ Nursing care plans address all the patient's needs in behavioral terms

◆ The nursing interventions implemented to achieve the nursing care goals fall under one of three categories

▶ Dependent actions follow a physician's order

▶ Independent actions provide individual, group, or family therapy

▶ Interdependent actions include referring specific areas of patient need, such as psychological testing, to another mental health team member

◆ Evaluation of care is continuous and includes the patient as an equal participant

■ The patient's reactions to the nursing care given validate the nursing interventions

■ Nursing implications of the nursing model

◆ The patient's needs direct the therapeutic relationship

◆ The nursing process is the basis for providing care

◆ Qualified psychiatric and mental health nurses provide individual and group psychotherapy

◆ The patient's reaction to nursing interventions guides future interventions

◆ The nurse provides holistic care, using the services of other disciplines as needed

❖ Behavioral model

■ This theory proposes that all behavior, including mental illness, is learned

■ Unlike other theoretical models, which focus on the patient's emotions, behavioral theory focuses on the patient's actions

■ Behavioral theorists, such as Skinner, Wolpe, and Eysenck, believe that by focusing on the patient's observed behavior, practitioners can use a strict scientific approach to study a therapy's effectiveness

■ Behavioral theory holds the following basic premises

◆ There's no such thing as a defect in the personality structure

◆ Behavior that's rewarded will persist, whether the behavior is good or bad

◆ Unwanted behaviors can be eliminated through negative sanctions such as punishment

◆ Desired behaviors can be learned through positive sanctions such as rewards

◆ Diagnostic labels are irrelevant; the focus of treatment is the behavior that requires change

■ Behavior can be changed through behavior modification (see "Behavior therapy," chapter 10, page 105)

■ Nursing implications of the behavioral model

◆ People can learn to behave in socially desirable ways

◆ The behavioral approach can be used with different personality types

◆ Consistency is important; failure to adhere to the treatment plan guarantees failure

◆ The patient's behavior (not pathology) is the focus of treatment

◆ Behavioral theory can be easily applied

❖ Medical model

■ Disease is the cause of deviant behavior

■ The medical model focuses on diagnosis and treatment of the disease

■ Curing the disease restores normal behavior

■ Modern psychiatry is dominated by adherents to the medical model

■ Medical interventions to cure mental disease include:

◆ *Somatic therapy* — electroconvulsive and drug therapy

◆ *Interpersonal therapy* — psychoanalysis and psychotherapy

■ Therapists adjust treatment protocols based on the patient's somatic response

■ Application of the medical model to mental illness has led to the identification of neurochemicals (such as enkephalins, serotonin, dopamine, and norepinephrine) as possible causes of deviant behavior

■ The medical model accepts socioenvironmental influences as potential causes of deviant behavior

◆ Social isolation, loneliness, and residence in an area associated with heavy drug use can cause a person to use drugs

◆ Working or living in an environment that exposes a person to high levels of carcinogens can cause disease

■ A central tenet of the medical model is the physician's control over the patient's therapy

■ Patients are expected to admit their sickness, conform to a treatment plan, and get well

■ Nursing implications of the medical model

◆ The treatment of disease is based on the patient's history and present condition, diagnosis, and laboratory studies

◆ The physician prescribes treatment and leads the treatment team

◆ Nurses and members of other health care disciplines are used in treatment when their expertise is required

◆ Interpersonal relations focus on the physician and the patient

❖ Communication models

■ Communication theory postulates that all human behavior is a form of communication

■ The meaning of the behavior depends on the clarity of communication between sender and receiver

■ Unclear communication produces anxiety, which results in behavioral deviation

■ Three communication models are widely accepted

◆ Berne's *transactional analysis* holds that communication is a unit called a transaction

▶ A transaction that's sent creates a complementary transaction when it's received and responded to by the receiver

▶ Communication occurs on three levels: parent, child, and adult

▶ When sender and receiver communicate on the same level, communication is referred to as a complementary transaction

▶ When transactions become crossed, the receiver responds differently than the sender expects and communication disruptions develop

◆ Bandler's and Grindler's *neurolinguistic programming* focuses on word choices and nonverbal communication

▶ People develop sensory channels (auditory, visual, kinesthetic) through which they receive communication

▶ Because they form a preference for one channel, communication harmony is established when both the sender and the receiver use the same channel

▶ Nonverbal communication (body language, speech pattern) is sent and received during any communication

◆ Watzlawick's *pragmatics of communication* holds that behavioral deviation results from disrupted communication patterns (noncommunication, lack of congruency in communication, imperviousness, and punctuation discrepancies)

■ Observing communication patterns can enhance understanding of behavioral disruptions

■ Nursing implications of the communication model

◆ The communication pattern used with individuals, families, and social and work groups identifies the cause of behavioral deviation

◆ Improving communication improves behavior

◆ The nurse teaches the patient effective communication techniques

◆ Effective communication by the patient should be reinforced

◆ Eliminating behavioral deviation requires the patient to participate in analyzing communication and in accepting responsibility for developing different communication styles

❖ Humanistic model

- Maslow, an American psychologist, has been credited with founding humanistic psychology
- Maslow is best known for describing a hierarchy of needs to understand human behavior
  - ◆ Physiologic survival
    - ▶ People at this most basic level are struggling for survival; working to obtain food, oxygen, and rest; and maintaining physiologic stability consume their energies
    - ▶ People who demonstrate behaviors that focus solely on these needs may have compromised health states
    - ▶ If these basic needs go unmet, the person could die; meeting them only partially causes personal discomfort
  - ◆ Safety, security, and self-preservation
    - ▶ Satisfying these needs is important to provide structure, predictability, and protection to the person's life
    - ▶ If these needs are unmet, the person will experience separation anxiety and fear of self-harm
  - ◆ Love and belonging
    - ▶ Being part of social groups and organizations allows a person to develop mutually fulfilling relationships
    - ▶ The person whose need for love and belonging is unmet will exhibit loneliness and experience feelings of alienation
  - ◆ Esteem and recognition
    - ▶ The person must feel like a worthwhile, contributing member of society; giving service to one's professional organization, serving on community boards, and appreciating one's own uniqueness are mechanisms for meeting this need
    - ▶ If the need for esteem and recognition goes unfilled, feelings of inferiority and helplessness will result
  - ◆ Self-actualization
    - ▶ To be self-actualized is to be self-fulfilled; people who know who they are, appreciate what they can do, face life's challenges confidently, have realistic expectations of themselves and others, and have a healthy sense of humor are self-actualized
    - ▶ If self-actualization needs go unmet, the person will experience loss of self-esteem and self-confidence
  - ◆ The aesthetic needs for truth, harmony, beauty, and spirituality
    - ▶ People who have become self-actualized will seek these needs
    - ▶ Frustration of these needs can result in dissatisfaction and restlessness
- Maslow believed that it was important to study people who are well adjusted, not just people who are maladjusted
- Maslow believed, unlike the behaviorists, that people are in control of their own behavioral choices, which are determined by underlying values rather than the external environment

■ Nursing implications of the humanistic model
  ◆ Lower-level needs must be met before higher-level needs can emerge
  ◆ Nurses must do a needs assessment, which enables them to determine appropriate intervention strategies for assisting patients to meet unmet needs
  ◆ People can choose to fulfill unmet needs but sometimes require assistance

❖ Change theories

■ Lewin's theory
  ◆ Behavior is a dynamic relationship between forces that work in opposite directions; these forces must be analyzed in order to facilitate change in the patient's behavior
    ▶ *Driving forces* facilitate change because they move participants in a desired direction
    ▶ *Restraining forces* interfere with change
  ◆ Change can be achieved only if there's an imbalance between the driving and restraining forces
  ◆ Change occurs via a three-step process
    ▶ Unfreezing
      • The patient's existing state of equilibrium is disturbed (this motivates the patient by preparing him for change)
      • The patient recognizes the need for change and builds trust
      • The nurse engages the patient in the process of identifying the problem and finding potential solutions
    ▶ Moving
      • The patient is moved to a new level of equilibrium (the patient is assisted in viewing the problem from a new perspective and agrees that the current status quo isn't beneficial)
      • The patient identifies with a practitioner who supports the change that is stimulated
      • The patient is encouraged to analyze his current behavior patterns in order to make the change
    ▶ Refreezing
      • The patient is frozen at a new level
      • New patterns of behavior are reinforced with formal and informal mechanisms, such as policies and hierarchy channels
■ Lippit's theory
  ◆ This theory focuses on the nurse's role as the change agent rather than the change itself
  ◆ There is a seven-step process for creating change
    ▶ *Diagnose the problem* — collecting data from key people assists in identifying the problem

▶ *Assess the patient's motivation and capacity for change*—assessing the resources and constraints and analyzing the organizational structure and function help determine the capacity for change

▶ *Assess the change agent's motivation and resources*—this is a self-assessment phase that's crucial for commitment to the proposed change; motivation, knowledge base, skills, and resources are all considered

▶ *Select progressive change objects*—a plan of action is developed, outcome criteria are established, and specific strategies are selected

▶ *Choose a change-agent role*—the role selected may include expert, consultant, teacher, or group facilitator

▶ *Maintain the change*—essential components of this phase include communication, feedback, revisions, and coordination; the change agent may need to provide support during this time

▶ *Terminate the helping relationship*—the change agent gradually withdraws from the process as the change becomes institutionalized

Review questions

1. A 4-year-old boy is struggling with whether to take a cookie out of the cookie jar without his mother's permission. Which of Freud's personality structures is activated in this situation?

○ **A.** Id

○ **B.** Ego

○ **C.** Superego

○ **D.** Id and superego

Correct answer: C The superego begins to develop at age 3 and houses one's conscience or sense of right and wrong. The id is present at birth and functions on needs, drives, and wishes. The ego begins to form between 4 and 5 months of age and mediates with the id and external reality.

2. A woman is called to the emergency department. The nurse tells her that her husband has been in an automobile accident and is in critical condition. The woman becomes so upset and anxious that she feels nauseous, begins to hyperventilate, and has to urinate frequently. According to Peplau, which level of anxiety is the woman experiencing?

○ **A.** Mild

○ **B.** Moderate

○ **C.** Severe

○ **D.** Panic

Correct answer: C Severe anxiety encompasses the symptoms outlined. Mild anxiety is a motivator and doesn't result in the symptoms described. Moderate anxiety is less intense in symptoms, and panic levels of anxiety are paralyzing in terms of functioning.

3. The nurse is working with a bipolar patient who has increased activity, difficulty focusing on tasks, and decreased ability to concentrate. The patient can't sit still for more than 5 minutes at a time and has lost 10 lb (4.5 kg) since her admission to the hospital. According to Maslow's hierarchy, which of the following levels of need should the nurse help the patient achieve?

○ **A.** Physiological survival

○ **B.** Safety, security, self preservation

○ **C.** Esteem and recognition

○ **D.** Self-actualization

Correct answer: A Physiological survival includes meeting basic needs, such as obtaining food, rest, and water. All other levels can be satisfied only after the physiological needs are met.

4. A mother tells her 6-year-old daughter that she can't have dessert because she didn't finish her supper. What theoretical model is the mother using?

○ **A.** Psychoanalytic

○ **B.** Behavioral

○ **C.** Social

○ **D.** Medical

Correct answer: B The mother is using the behavioral model, which focuses on rewarding positive behaviors and eliminating unwanted behaviors through negative sanctions such as punishment.

5. A woman has difficulty expressing her thoughts and feelings to her husband. The nurse is working with the woman on assertive communication. Which of the following models is the nurse most likely utilizing with this patient?

○ **A.** Behavioral model

○ **B.** Medical model

○ **C.** Communication model

○ **D.** Humanistic model

Correct answer: C The nurse is most likely using the communication model because it focuses on analyzing human interactions and teaching effective communication skills.

Nursing research

❖ Overview

■ Research is a systematic, logical, and empirical inquiry into the possible relationships among particular phenomena

■ It's a scientific method for gathering, analyzing, and disseminating new information

■ Nursing research is that scientific method applied to the study of any nursing problem, with the goal of expanding the theoretical basis of nursing through the discovery of new knowledge

■ Understanding the steps and techniques that researchers use enables the nurse to participate actively in research that benefits nursing

■ The nurse is then better able to judge the soundness of research findings before applying them in the clinical setting

■ All nurses are mandated by nursing practice standards (See Appendix A, Standards of psychiatric and mental health clinical nursing practice.) to contribute to the growth of nursing knowledge by participating in the research process

■ Nursing research links nursing theory, education, and practice

■ Nursing theory is developed from practice and must be validated by research to be useful

■ Research can be descriptive, explanatory, or predictive

◆ *Descriptive research* obtains accurate information about the phenomenon under investigation; the investigator observes, describes, and classifies

◆ *Explanatory research* attempts to understand the relationship among the phenomena under investigation; the investigator explains observed events and their relationships to each other and to outside influences

◆ *Predictive research* uses statistical measures to forecast the relationships among phenomena

❖ Types of nursing research

■ Nurses use several methods to identify, gather, and analyze information

■ The method selected depends on which questions the nurse-researcher wants to ask

■ The investigator uses two broad types of nursing research: quantitative and qualitative

◆ *Quantitative nursing research* involves the systematic collection of data in numerical format, under strict researcher control, and the analysis of that data in order to describe, explain, or predict a particular phenomenon (for example, research describing the views held by adolescents, parents, and school personnel toward adolescent suicide)

◆ *Qualitative nursing research* involves the systematic collection and analysis of subjective information (with attempts to minimize researcher-imposed control in the absence of statistical methodology) in order to understand the depth of a particular phenomenon (for example, research exploring the experience of survival and bereavement after a loved one dies from acquired immunodeficiency syndrome [AIDS])

■ Because many of the research questions that interest nurses are complex, some researchers believe that neither the qualitative nor the quantitative method of research alone is sufficient

■ Increasing numbers of research studies are using both qualitative and quantitative methods (for example, a study of the psychological distress that can result from using a computer versus a pen and pencil for testing purposes)

❖ **Phases of nursing research**

■ *Gathering data,* the first major phase of nursing research, requires eight essential steps

◆ Consider research ethics and the rights of human subjects

❯ Before gathering research data, the nurse must understand the risks and benefits inherent in any research study

❯ Because most nursing research involves human subjects, the nurse must carefully consider the procedures used in order to protect the rights of those subjects

❯ Subjects have the right to refuse participation in the study, and those who volunteer have the right to review and sign an informed consent before research begins

❯ Subjects have the right to privacy, confidentiality, and fair treatment

❯ The American Nurses Association's "Human Rights Guidelines for Nurses in Clinical and Other Research" addresses research problems of particular concern to nurses

◆ Select a research problem

❯ A thorough research investigator spends considerable time selecting and defining a problem for study because the problem provides direction for the study

❯ Practical experience, scientific literature, and untested theory are all rich sources of research problems (for example, a nurse working with patients with AIDS might want to examine what it's like to have the disease; another nurse, working with the same population, might want to explore whether nurses' attitudes toward patients with AIDS influence the patients' emotional well-being)

◆ Identify the research question

  ▶ Although nurses may raise many legitimate questions about their practice, not all these questions can be reasonably pursued through research

  ▶ Before selecting the research question, the nurse must consider four criteria

   • The research question should be of sufficient significance to nursing and health care

   • Researching the question should be feasible (inadequate time or funding, unavailability of subjects, lack of proper equipment, and ethical concerns are among the numerous problems that can hinder research)

   • Knowledge gained from the research must outweigh the cost of obtaining it

   • The topic should hold the researcher's interest over the duration of the study

◆ State the research problem

  ▶ The problem must be worded clearly to guide the design of the study

  ▶ Experienced researchers differ as to whether the problem should be phrased as a statement or as a question

  ▶ It must specify the subject to be studied, along with key variables amenable to observation or measurement

   • Variables are the properties that differ from one subject to another

   • Dependent variables are the concepts that the researcher wants to explain or predict; commonly referred to as "the consequence," they're assumed to vary with changes in the independent variables

   • Independent (or antecedent) variables presumably affect the dependent variables; the researcher typically manipulates these variables in an experimental study

   • Variables aren't inherently dependent or independent (for example, alcoholism may be the dependent variable in a study of factors that predict alcoholism and an independent variable in a study of domestic violence)

   • Variables should be placed in a theoretical or conceptual context

  ▶ The scope of the problem must be precisely delineated so that the research direction is evident (for example, "What's the relationship between perception of autonomy and job satisfaction in a group of psychiatric nurses?" The independent variable [perception of autonomy] is presumed to affect the dependent variable [job satisfaction] of a specific population [psychiatric nurses])

◆ Review the literature
  ▶ All research studies demand a thorough review of the appropriate literature
  ▶ Timing of the review depends on the nature of the research question
    • In most quantitative studies, the researcher conducts a thorough review before collecting data to identify potential gaps in the literature and to examine the approaches others have taken in studying a particular problem
    • In qualitative studies, the researcher commonly collects data before an extensive literature review to minimize researcher bias
  ▶ The review must include data-based and conceptual literature
    • Data-based literature addresses the problem of interest
    • Conceptual literature addresses underlying theories of the problem
  ▶ The review should also encompass statistics, research findings, methods and procedures, opinions, beliefs, and clinical impressions and situations relevant to the study
  ▶ The review should include primary and secondary research sources
    • Primary sources are articles written by the investigator who conducted the research or proposed the theory
    • Secondary sources are reviews of primary sources; although they frequently prove useful in supplying additional references on the topic, secondary sources shouldn't be substituted for primary sources because they provide less detail and may expose the researcher to the second author's bias
◆ Develop a theory (theoretical framework)
  ▶ A theory is a statement that attempts to describe, explain, or predict some phenomenon
  ▶ It guides the researcher in separating critical and necessary factors or relationships from accidental ones
  ▶ A theory consists of the abstract concepts being studied (such as health, anxiety, stress, or pain) and a set of propositions that depict the relationships among the concepts
  ▶ A theory is built inductively from research and then tested deductively by research
    • Most qualitative research is inductive; researchers primarily use it to develop a theory
    • Most quantitative research is deductive; researchers primarily use it to test a theory
◆ Develop a hypothesis
  ▶ After stating the problem, reviewing the literature, and choosing a theoretical framework, the researcher formulates a hypothesis
  ▶ The hypothesis is derived from the theory and serves as a prediction or preliminary explanation of the relationships among variables

◗ Written as a declarative statement, it delineates the relationship between at least two variables, one dependent and one independent

◗ A hypothesis can be simple or complex, formulated directionally or nondirectionally

• A *simple hypothesis* expresses an expected relationship between one independent and one dependent variable (for example, "There's a relationship between perception of autonomy and job satisfaction among psychiatric nurses")

• A *complex hypothesis* expresses a relationship between two or more independent variables and two or more dependent variables (for example, "A relationship exists between level of education, perception of autonomy, and job satisfaction among psychiatric nurses")

• In a *directionally formulated hypothesis*, the researcher predicts the nature as well as the existence of a relationship (for example, "Nurses with higher education and more work autonomy will experience greater job satisfaction than nurses with less education and less work autonomy")

• In a *nondirectionally formulated hypothesis*, the researcher predicts the existence of a relationship only (see the first example above)

◗ Hypotheses are classified as either research or statistical hypotheses

• A research hypothesis expresses a relationship between the independent and the dependent variables (the examples above are research hypotheses)

• Conversely, a statistical (or null) hypothesis states that no relationship exists between the independent and dependent variables

◆ Build the research design

◗ The design is a framework that the researcher creates, a set of instructions that tell the researcher how to collect and analyze data in order to answer a specified research problem

◗ The problem statement, literature review, theory, and hypothesis all contribute to this design

■ *Manipulating data,* the second major phase of nursing research, involves measurement and analysis of quantitative and qualitative information

◆ In many quantitative studies, nurse researchers use instruments or tools to measure subjective psychosocial concepts (such as attitudes, stress, and social support systems) that can't otherwise be measured

◗ Before using any tool, the nurse must evaluate its validity and reliability

• *Validity* is the extent to which an instrument measures what it claims to measure (for example, does a tool that claims to measure introversion or extroversion really measure those traits?)

• There are three types of validity: criterion, content, and construct

- *Reliability* is the extent to which an instrument yields the same results on repeated trials
- The researcher uses four methods — retest, split-half, alternative form, and coefficient alpha — to evaluate an instrument's reliability

▶ When manipulating quantitative data, the researcher uses statistical and sampling techniques to assign numerical values to what has been measured

- *Statistical techniques* enable the researcher to analyze resulting numerical values
  - Scales are commonly used to express all possible values of a given measurement
  - As an example, job satisfaction might be rated on a scale of 1 (least satisfied) to 6 (most satisfied)
- *Sampling* is the process of selecting a portion of a population to represent the entire group
  - Probability sampling uses random selection so that every member of the population has an equal chance of being selected
  - Commonly used probability methods include simple random, stratified random, cluster, and systematic sampling
  - Probability sampling, the basis of most statistical testing, avoids bias but can be costly and inconvenient
  - Nonprobability sampling uses arbitrary judgment or defined characteristics of the population as samples
  - Samples of convenience and selections by quota are examples of nonprobability samples
  - The researcher should use as large a sample as possible, given the constraints of the study

▶ When the data have been collected in a quantitative study, researchers use statistical analysis to make sense out of the findings; the analysis can be descriptive or inferential

- *Descriptive statistics* organize, summarize, and present information coherently (for instance, measurement of the mean, median, mode, and standard deviation of the sample)
- *Inferential statistics* make inferences about populations based on the samples taken from them, using the logic that chance is the only thing that produces variations in the study
  - Inferential statistics test the hypothesis
  - Examples of inferential statistical tests include t-tests, F tests, chi-square, ANOVA, and regression analysis

◆ Qualitative research focuses on human subjectivity, using inductive reasoning, natural settings, descriptive data, and process-oriented questions; examples include case studies, grounded theory, phenomenology, and ethnography

▶ *Case studies* provide an in-depth examination of one or more subjects to develop a profile of what happens to an individual subject in a given situation

▶ *Grounded theory* is inductively derived from studying the phenomenon it represents
  • The research question in a grounded study identifies the phenomenon to be studied (for example, "How do nurse psychotherapists experience the termination phase of therapy?")
  • The research is a continual process of making comparisons and asking questions
  • Data are collected (usually by interview and field notes) and analyzed until the researcher reaches a saturation point
▶ *Phenomenology* explores the experience of life as it's lived (for example, "What's the experience of living with AIDS?"); analysis then focuses on abstracting the essential meaning of the experience
▶ *Ethnography* examines the norms, values, and knowledge of a specific culture (for example, "What does self-care mean in the culture of the intensive care unit?")
  • In this type of study, the researcher uses interviews, participant observations, and records to focus on the sample's culture rather than the individual experience
  • Data analysis proceeds concurrently with data collection
■ *Reporting data*, the final phase of nursing research, uses descriptive or inferential statistical methods to reveal the results of the study
  ◆ The final research report must identify the methods used to analyze data (such as the computer software used)
  ◆ The report may use inferential statistics to predict whether relationships in the study sample are likely to occur in the population at large
    ▶ A report that uses these statistics should also include information needed to assess the findings
    ▶ Such information includes the statistical test used (for example, t-test, ANOVA), the magnitude of the test, the degrees of freedom, the probability level, and the direction of the effect found
  ◆ The researcher should evaluate the results and interpret the implications according to the original hypothesis, including a statement that clearly expresses whether the results are statistically significant (that is, whether they do or don't support the hypothesis)
  ◆ The report should clearly and thoroughly present the researcher's conclusions about the accuracy and meaning of the results
  ◆ The report also should address the importance of the study, commenting on the applicability of findings to the general population, implications for nursing practice, and directions for future research

❖ **The role of nurses in nursing research**
  ■ The use of research findings enables the nurse to provide the best possible nursing care
  ■ Nurses can participate in research and document the unique role nursing plays in the health care system
  ■ Through participation in research studies, the nurse contributes toward the construction of a scientific knowledge base for nursing practice

■ The nurse can implement research findings that demonstrate strategies to decrease health care costs

❖ **The use of research findings in nursing practice**
■ As a health care provider, the nurse evaluates the relevance of research findings and can apply that knowledge in practice
■ Because the nurse is aware of a significant number of studies with common sample characteristics, the nurse can implement a similar study in the nurse's own clinical setting or environment
■ Information from research studies can be reviewed by the nurse for its applicability to specific client populations; further studies can be generated to validate the application of the research information
■ Consistent findings in nursing research can warrant changes to current standards of clinical practice

Review questions

1. Which of the following is an example of a primary source for a nursing research study?

   ○ **A.** A summary of research that has been performed on the study topic

   ○ **B.** The retrieval mechanism used to locate the actual statistical research information

   ○ **C.** An index that directs the reader to the research study's methodology

   ○ **D.** A description of the study written by the researcher who conducted the study

   Correct answer: D   Primary sources are the articles written by the person who performs the actual research study.

2. Which of the following is the most important reason for doing a literature review before constructing a research study?

   ○ **A.** The research design can be copied from another study.

   ○ **B.** Helpful information on demographic instrument development could be uncovered.

   ○ **C.** Existing knowledge about the identified problem can be found.

   ○ **D.** A determination of the study's feasibility could be extrapolated.

   Correct answer: C   A review of the literature includes the available theoretical knowledge and published research on the topic to be investigated.

3. What does nursing research contribute to the advancement of profession-al nursing practice?

   ○ **A.** Investigation of theoretical models

   ○ **B.** Expansion of scientific knowledge

   ○ **C.** Preparation of proficient clinicians

   ○ **D.** Foundation of collaborative activity

Correct answer: B Nursing research is the scientific process used to collect and disseminate knowledge about particular phenomena. The research process contributes to the growth of nursing knowledge.

4. What contribution does qualitative research make to professional nursing practice?

   ○ **A.** Clinical experiences are processed and interventions are established.

   ○ **B.** Knowledge is advanced and theories are further developed.

   ○ **C.** Explanations for quantitative research findings are reinforced.

   ○ **D.** Outcomes of care plans are made observable and measurable.

Correct answer: B Qualitative research is used to examine a phenomenon of interest when limited information is known about the concept, its relationship patterns, and theoretical formulations.

5. The following hypothesis is to be tested: Female adolescents who were abused as children are at greater risk for depression and suicide than adolescents with no history of abuse. What's the independent variable?

   ○ **A.** Female gender

   ○ **B.** History of abuse

   ○ **C.** Risk of depression

   ○ **D.** Abused adolescents

Correct answer: B The independent variable is the variable that's believed to influence the dependent variable. In this hypothesis, the history of abuse is believed to influence a female adolescent's risk for depression and suicide.

Therapeutic communication

❖ Overview

- ■ Communication is the process by which people transmit ideas and feelings to one another
- ■ According to communication theory, behavior is a form of communication that's influenced by a person's culture and experiences
- ■ All behavior is communication and all communication affects behavior
- ■ Communication can be verbal or nonverbal, constructive or destructive
  - ◆ Verbal communication is the use of spoken or written language to transmit information; it includes how words and phrases are used to convey meaning
  - ◆ Nonverbal communication is the use of physical movement to convey messages; besides body language, nonverbal communication can include such disparate elements as voice sounds (groans or grunts to convey displeasure) and hair and clothing styles (to promote a certain image)
  - ◆ Constructive communication from the sender confirms the receiver's importance and promotes self-esteem
  - ◆ Destructive communication from the sender belittles the receiver's importance and diminishes self-esteem
- ■ Therapeutic communication is an interactive process that occurs between the patient and the health professional; meaningful and intense, it focuses solely on the patient's problems (See *Characteristics of social and therapeutic relationships,* page 62.)
  - ◆ Therapeutic communication is the foundation for establishing a therapeutic nurse-patient relationship
  - ◆ Therapeutic communication requires the nurse to select words and phrases carefully in order to establish a dialogue with the patient
  - ◆ The purpose of therapeutic communication is to elicit information about a patient's needs, feelings, and ideas so the nurse can understand the patient's problems and develop interventions that strengthen a patient's insight and self-control

Characteristics of social and therapeutic relationships

In an effective nurse-patient relationship, the psychiatric and mental health nurse uses therapeutic communication to shed light on and promote healthy changes in the patient's behavior. The chart below contrasts important differences between a therapeutic relationship and a purely social one.

Social relationship	Therapeutic relationship
Focuses on mutual sharing, with each participant giving and taking	Focuses on the patient, with the nurse giving and the patient taking
Promotes mutual pleasure	Promotes patient healing
Has no time constraints	Is time-limited
Doesn't involve a contract	Involves a contract between the nurse and the patient
Doesn't require the participants to examine their behavior or to possess a specialized knowledge base	Requires the nurse to have a profound understanding of the nurse-patient relationship and to examine each participant's behavior from a theoretical perspective

❖ **Principles of therapeutic communication**
  ■ Genuineness
    ◆ The nurse must display a sincere interest in the patient and the patient's problems by using consistent words and actions
    ◆ Such authenticity promotes openness, self-acceptance, and personal freedom in the patient
  ■ Respect
    ◆ The nurse must have an unconditional positive regard for the patient
    ◆ Nonjudgmental acceptance of the patient's ideas and beliefs communicates the nurse's willingness to work with the patient
  ■ Honesty
    ◆ A consistent, open, and frank approach promotes authenticity in the nurse-patient relationship
    ◆ The patient will be more likely to accept and trust a nurse who is honest and forthright
  ■ Concreteness
    ◆ The nurse should use clear, specific, concrete language rather than abstractions when communicating with the patient
    ◆ Concreteness keeps the nurse's responses close to the patient's experiences and feelings, fosters the nurse's accuracy of understanding, and encourages the patient to focus on specific problem areas
  ■ Assistance

◆ The nurse must exhibit a willing commitment to the nurse-patient relationship

◆ A willing commitment conveys that the nurse has something of value to offer the patient

■ Protection

◆ The patient must feel safe from confrontations with threatening forces (either self-harm or harm from others)

◆ Ensuring the patient's safety promotes a successful relationship

■ Permission

◆ The patient who feels free to explore new ways of dealing with past problems builds autonomy

◆ The patient's learning to try alternative behaviors is central to eliminating the patient's problems

❖ Blocks to constructive communication

■ Giving advice prevents the patient from forming independent conclusions and promotes dependence

■ Providing false reassurance may inhibit the patient from disclosing true feelings

■ Asking "why" questions yields scant information and may overwhelm the patient, leading to stress and withdrawal; cause the patient to become defensive; or force the patient to answer to please the nurse, whether or not the response makes sense

■ Using emotionally charged language may intimidate or shame the patient and lead to withdrawal

■ Straying from the patient's agenda shifts the thrust of the nurse-patient interaction away from the patient's concerns; a patient who detects the nurse's disinterest will feel unimportant and demeaned

■ Using clichés shows a poor understanding of the patient's uniqueness and conveys unwillingness to get involved, possibly leading the patient to feel unheard, alone, discounted, and misunderstood

■ Delivering double messages (such as contradicting a verbal message with a nonverbal one) confuses the patient, who may become indecisive, anxious, and withdrawn

■ Lecturing the patient inhibits problem solving and suggests that the patient is incapable of independent thinking

❖ Requirements for therapeutic communication

■ Maintain privacy

◆ The patient may be embarrassed or afraid to disclose personal and private information

◆ Fear that the conversation will be overheard or revealed can discourage the patient from being open and honest

■ Preserve the patient's self-esteem

◆ Conveying an unconditional and positive regard for the patient promotes self-disclosure

◆ The patient needs to feel valued and respected regardless of behavior or physical appearance
■ Choose words carefully
◆ Language influences the therapeutic atmosphere
◆ The nurse should avoid judgmental, demeaning, or threatening terms
■ Ask questions in a precise order
◆ First, ask how the patient would describe the situation or problem
▶ This question is emotionally neutral and elicits important data
▶ The question immediately involves the patient and conveys the nurse's interest
◆ Next, ask what the patient thinks about the situation or problem
▶ The patient's thoughts provide assessment data
▶ Soliciting the patient's interpretation maintains involvement
◆ Finally, ask how the patient feels about the situation or problem
▶ Sharing feelings may be frightening to the patient, especially when the interview begins; covering this essential assessment step later in the interview commonly elicits useful information
▶ The nurse should accept and evaluate the patient's feelings nonjudgmentally

❖ **Techniques of therapeutic communication**
■ Listening
◆ Focusing intently on the patient enables the nurse to hear and analyze everything the patient is saying
◆ Such attention can alert the nurse to the patient's communication patterns
■ Restating
◆ Succinct rephrasing helps ensure the nurse's understanding and emphasizes important points in the patient's message
◆ Rephrasing also confirms the nurse's attention, interest, and empathy and may promote further disclosure
■ Using broad openings
◆ General statements or questions that begin with what, when, where and how (such as "where were you when you felt anxious?") to initiate a conversation encourage the patient to raise any subject
◆ General questions also focus the discussion on the patient and demonstrate the nurse's willingness to interact
■ Clarifying
◆ Attempting to put a patient's confusing or vague message into words or asking the patient what he or she means demonstrates the nurse's desire to understand what the patient is saying
◆ Attempting to clarify a vague message can also elicit more precise information crucial to the patient's recovery
■ Confrontation

◆ The confrontation technique calls attention to discrepancies the nurse perceives in a patient's communication patterns

◆ Discrepancies occur between the patient's expression of self-concept (who the patient is) and self-ideal (who the patient wants to be); between the patient's verbal and non-verbal expression; between the patient's self experience and the nurse's experience of the patient

◆ After confronting the patient with the discrepancy, the nurse waits for a response

■ Focusing

◆ Helping the patient expand on a topic of importance keeps the communication goal-directed

◆ Focusing on an important topic fosters the patient's self-control and helps avoid vague generalizations, thereby enabling the patient to accept responsibility for facing problems

■ Silence

◆ Refraining from making comments can have several benefits: it gives the patient time to think, talk, and gain insight into problems and permits the nurse to gather more information

◆ The nurse must use this technique judiciously, however, or else the patient may perceive the nurse's silence as disinterest or rejection

■ Suggesting (presenting alternatives for the patient to consider)

◆ Used during the working phase of the nurse-patient relationship, this technique can help the patient see previously untapped options

◆ When used correctly, the technique gives the patient the opportunity to explore the pros and cons of numerous choices

◆ Presenting alternatives must be used carefully to avoid directing the patient

■ Sharing perceptions

◆ In this technique, the nurse describes his or her understanding of the patient's feelings and then seeks corrective feedback from the patient

◆ This techniques also allows the patient to clarify any misperceptions and gives the nurse a better understanding of the patient's true feelings

■ Identifying themes

◆ In this technique, the nurse states the experiences, issues, or problems the patient discloses repeatedly during the interaction

◆ Use of this technique promotes patient exploration and understanding of problem areas

■ Reflecting

◆ In this technique, the nurse repeats the patient's ideas, feelings, questions, or content

◆ Reflecting helps show the nurse's understanding of the patient's communication

◆ Reflecting also imparts interest, empathy, and respect for the patient

❖ Guidelines for establishing therapeutic communication
- ■ Attend to the reality of the patient's experience
  - ◆ Focus on the patient's questions and feelings
  - ◆ Seek more data on the patient's perceptions and thoughts
- ■ Give the patient information
  - ◆ Explain what to expect from the staff
  - ◆ State the nursing unit's rules
  - ◆ Describe what's expected of the patient while on the unit
  - ◆ Identify who will give care
- ■ Empower the patient
  - ◆ Include the patient in care conferences
  - ◆ Ask the patient to contribute to care planning
  - ◆ Determine the patient's expectations
- ■ Anticipate the patient's needs
  - ◆ Begin discharge planning as soon as the patient enters the therapeutic environment
  - ◆ Provide privacy and personal space
  - ◆ Conserve the patient's energy to allow for healing
  - ◆ Provide diversional activities as the patient's energy level increases
- ■ Be accountable to the patient
  - ◆ Keep the patient informed about the care plan
  - ◆ Ask for the patient's input about care

Review questions

1. In which phase of the nurse-patient relationship would the nurse appropriately use the communication technique of confrontation?

- ○ **A.** Introduction
- ○ **B.** Orientation
- ○ **C.** Working
- ○ **D.** Termination

Correct answer: C   The nurse must first establish a working relationship with the patient so the patient trusts and accepts the nurse's feedback about discrepancies in behavior. Promoting patient insight is a task of the working relationship.

2. Which of the following actions would negate the principle of genuineness of the nurse?

- ○ **A.** The nurse smiles at a joke the patient has told.
- ○ **B.** The nurse shows unconditional positive regard.
- ○ **C.** The nurse's behavior is inconsistent with her words.
- ○ **D.** The nurse self-discloses.

Correct answer: C Genuineness and sincerity are demonstrated by consistency in words and actions.

3. Therapeutic communication differs from social communication in that therapeutic communication requires the nurse to do which of the following actions?

○ **A.** Limit activities with the patient to therapeutic endeavors.

○ **B.** Examine the patient's behavior from a theoretical perspective.

○ **C.** Focus on mutual sharing so as to not intimidate the patient.

○ **D.** Avoid setting expectations as a part of the contract.

Correct answer: B Examining the patient's behavior from a theoretical perspective is a professional obligation and has no place in a social interaction.

4. Using clichés in therapeutic communication leads the patient toward:

○ **A.** viewing the nurse as human.

○ **B.** accepting self as human.

○ **C.** self-disclosing.

○ **D.** feeling discounted.

Correct answer: D The use of clichés is commonly construed by the patient as the nurse's lack of understanding, involvement, and caring, and thus the patient may feel demeaned and discounted.

5. In assessing the patient, the nurse begins by asking questions that encourage the patient to describe problematic behaviors and situations. The next step is to elicit the patient's:

○ **A.** feelings about what has been described.

○ **B.** thoughts about what has been described.

○ **C.** possible solutions to the problem.

○ **D.** intent in sharing the description.

Correct answer: B Questions should be asked in a precise order, specifically from the most simple description to the more difficult disclosure of feelings. When the problem has been described, eliciting the patient's thoughts about the dilemmas provides further assessment data as well as the patient's interpretation of what has happened. Feelings, solutions, and articulating intent (why information is shared at a particular moment) are more complex processes, especially if the patient is highly anxious or out of touch with reality.

Legal aspects of nursing practice

❖ **Overview**
- Safe psychiatric and mental health nursing practice requires a basic understanding of the federal and state laws and regulations that affect nursing practice
- State laws that affect psychiatric and mental health nursing practice vary from state to state
- Nurses practicing psychiatric and mental health nursing should become familiar with the laws of the state in which they practice

❖ **Torts**
- A tort is a civil wrong
- It's a violation of a person's private rights that entitles the person who has been wronged to seek damages from the wrongdoer
- Unintentional torts (negligence) and intentional torts are two areas of tort liability that have an impact on psychiatric and mental health nursing practice
  - ◆ Unintentional torts (negligence)
    - ❭ For a psychiatric patient to recover damages for a claim against a nurse, four elements of nursing negligence must be present
      - • The nurse must owe the patient a duty of care
      - • The nurse must breach the duty of care
      - • The patient must suffer damages
      - • The nurse's breach of duty must be the cause of the patient's damages
    - ❭ Whether a psychiatric and mental health nurse owes a patient a duty of care depends on whether a nurse-patient relationship had been established
    - ❭ A psychiatric and mental health nurse owes a patient a duty to use that degree of knowledge and skill normally possessed by professional peers and to provide nursing services that meet accepted standards of psychiatric and mental health nursing practice
    - ❭ A psychiatric and mental health nurse breaches the duty owed a patient if the nursing care provided fails to meet the standards
      - • A standard of care is generally measured by comparing the actions (or inactions) of the psychiatric and mental health nurse with the actions (or inactions) of a reasonable and prudent psychi-

atric and mental health nurse functioning under the same or similar circumstances

- A standard of care can be derived from the following sources:
  - The Nurse Practice Act and concomitant regulations of the state in which the psychiatric and mental health nurse practices
  - "Code for Nurses with Interpretive Statements," by the American Nurses Association (ANA)
  - The ANA's "Standards of Psychiatric and Mental Health Nursing Practice"
  - "Consolidated Standards Manual for Child, Adolescent and Adult Psychiatric, Alcoholism and Drug Abuse Facilities," by the Joint Commission on Accreditation of Healthcare Organizations
  - Professional journals such as *Journal of Psychosocial Nursing and Mental Health Services,* the official journal of the American Psychiatric Nurses Association
  - Experts in psychiatric and mental health nursing

▶ An injured patient may file a lawsuit against a psychiatric and mental health nurse to seek compensatory damages for pain, suffering, and economic losses (such as medical expenses and lost wages) resulting from the nurse's negligence

▶ Common negligence allegations brought against psychiatric and mental health nurses include failure to monitor for changes in a patient's condition, abandonment (leaving a patient unattended), medication errors, negligent supervision of staff, and failure to ensure patient safety

◆ Intentional torts

▶ Unlike negligent acts, which suggest unintended carelessness, intentional torts signify an intent to commit the act

▶ Intentional torts also differ from negligence in that the patient need not show proof of damages; the patient may be entitled to punitive damages (in addition to compensatory damages), which serves to punish the wrongdoer

▶ Common allegations against psychiatric and mental health nurses for committing intentional torts include the following:

- Invasion of privacy commonly arises in conjunction with treating a psychiatric patient without obtaining informed consent
- False imprisonment commonly arises in conjunction with involuntary confinement and the use of restraints or seclusion
- Battery or assault charges usually involve physical contact with a patient (or threats to do so) without the patient's consent
- Breach of confidentiality

▶ Psychiatric and mental health nurses can prevent or limit claims of negligence and intentional torts in several ways

- Provide safe nursing practice in accordance with the profession's standards of care (the best line of defense is prevention)

● Ensure adequate documentation in the patient's record
● Understand the doctrine of assumption of risk: a patient who refuses treatment knowing that the refusal could cause harm to self or others assumes the risk of harm, and the nurse cannot be held liable for the patient's refusal
● Understand the doctrine of comparative negligence
  – If a nurse and a patient are both found negligent, the damages the patient seeks to recover from the nurse may be reduced
  – If the nurse's employer or another health care provider is found negligent along with the nurse, the employer or other health care provider must pay a portion of the damages
● Become familiar with governmental immunity statutes, which may prohibit a patient from suing a psychiatric and mental health nurse employed by a state or federal agency or institution

❖ **Informed consent**
■ All psychiatric patients have the right to determine the treatment they will accept or reject
■ This right is encompassed in the legal doctrine of informed consent, which requires the psychiatric patient to be advised of the contemplated treatment plan
■ Health care personnel are required to obtain the patient's consent before treatment
■ The doctrine of informed consent is derived from common law and constitutional law
  ◆ Common law
    ▶ Common law is based on prior judicial opinions
    ▶ Common law recognizes a patient's right to self-determination, the right to determine what shall be done to one's body
  ◆ Constitutional law
    ▶ The United States and individual state constitutions guarantee people certain fundamental rights; among them is the right of privacy
    ▶ Courts have interpreted the constitutional right of privacy to include the right to accept or reject medical treatment
■ The right to informed consent isn't an exclusive right; it must be balanced against certain state interests
  ◆ Each state has an interest in preserving life, preventing suicide, and protecting innocent third parties
  ◆ If a psychiatric patient threatens self-harm or harm to others, a state's interest in preventing such actions could outweigh the patient's right to refuse treatment
  ◆ The patient would then be compelled to undergo treatment despite a personal unwillingness
■ Certain information must be disclosed to a psychiatric patient in order to obtain informed consent

◆ The proposed treatment

◆ The material risks associated with the proposed treatment

◆ Alternative treatments available

◆ The material risks associated with the alternative treatments

◆ The consequences if treatment isn't rendered

■ Different states have different legal standards to determine whether informed consent was appropriately obtained

◆ Most states have adopted the "prudent patient" standard, which requires health care personnel to disclose the information a reasonable or prudent patient would need to know to give informed consent

◆ Some states subscribe to the professional standard, which requires health care personnel to disclose information that other reasonable and prudent health care personnel normally disclose to a patient to obtain informed consent

◆ The more stringent prudent patient standard is in keeping with the trends of expanding patients' rights and including patients in the health care decision-making process

■ Problems with obtaining adequate informed consent can arise in various circumstances in psychiatric settings

◆ Generally, minors cannot give informed consent because they haven't attained the age of legal capacity (18 in most states)

▶ The child's parent or legal guardian must provide the necessary consent

▶ Some state statutes contain exceptions that allow minors to give informed consent under certain circumstances (for example, if the minor is married or pregnant or is seeking treatment for drug use or drug dependency)

◆ An adult must have the capacity to make decisions in order to give informed consent

▶ Although an adult is presumed competent until proved incompetent in a court of law, a psychiatric patient whose mental competency is questionable may be presented for treatment

▶ Most state statutes provide procedures for these occasions, requiring a court hearing to determine whether a patient is competent and appointing a legal guardian, if necessary

▶ If a patient is deemed incompetent, informed consent must be obtained from a legal guardian

◆ The doctrine of informed consent also applies to patients who are committed either voluntarily or involuntarily to a mental health facility

◆ Commitment, whether voluntary or involuntary, doesn't mean that a patient is incompetent or that any rights have been forfeited

■ Certain exceptions permit psychiatric treatment without obtaining informed consent from a patient

◆ In an emergency (for example, if a psychiatric patient is found unconscious), consent to treatment will be implied

◆ Informed consent isn't needed if disclosure of the information necessary to obtain the consent would adversely affect the patient
■ The psychiatric and mental health nurse's role can vary in practice situations requiring informed consent
　◆ Generally, obtaining a patient's informed consent is the responsibility of the attending physician; the nurse commonly serves as a witness to the patient's signature on a consent form
　◆ If the nurse has reason to believe that the patient wasn't adequately informed or may lack the capacity to give informed consent, the nurse shouldn't permit the patient to sign the consent form; instead, the nurse should provide adequate information or contact the patient's guardian
　◆ In some situations, the psychiatric and mental health nurse may be required to obtain informed consent for nursing procedures, or a nurse may be required to carry out a physician's order that the patient is resisting; in either case, providing treatment that has been refused could expose the nurse to a lawsuit for invasion of privacy and for assault and battery
　◆ Even if informed consent was previously obtained, the patient may revoke it at any time

❖ **Confinement**
■ The psychiatric patient may be voluntarily admitted or involuntarily committed to a psychiatric facility
　◆ Voluntary admission is generally available to mentally ill adults whose mental health needs cannot be met without in-facility care or whose mental illness causes them to be dangerous to themselves, others, or property
　　▸ A patient is deemed dangerous if he or she has threatened or attempted suicide, is substantially likely to harm another, is unable to provide basic needs to such an extent that serious bodily harm will ensue, or is substantially likely to cause serious damage to property
　　▸ A patient who is voluntarily admitted has the right to be discharged under certain conditions (most states accept the following conditions; the nurse should consult applicable state laws before implementing voluntary discharge)
　　　• The request must be documented in the patient's chart
　　　• The patient must be discharged unless the facility seeks involuntary commitment (because the patient poses a danger to self, others, or property) and obtains a temporary court order to retain the patient pending a full hearing by a court
　　　• If a temporary court order to hold the patient isn't obtained within 2 days of the request to be discharged, the patient must be discharged
　◆ Involuntary commitment is required when a mentally ill adult is unwilling to be admitted voluntarily for treatment

▶ Specific statutory procedures must be followed to consummate involuntary commitment

▶ The determination permitting the involuntary commitment must be reviewed periodically

▶ Any mentally ill adult who is believed to need commitment will be assessed by a designated local mental health screening facility

▶ The patient can come alone, be referred by a family member, or be brought to the facility by a law enforcement officer

▶ The patient can be detained at the screening facility for 1 day for assessment and treatment

▶ When the patient is assessed by the screening facility, appropriate mental health services must be recommended for the patient

▶ If involuntary commitment is deemed necessary by the mental health staff, the patient will be committed to an appropriate facility as soon as possible, even if the patient objects to the confinement

▶ If there is no need for admission or commitment, the patient is referred to the appropriate clinic services

▶ A patient cannot be committed involuntarily unless the patient exhibits the same dangerous behavioral propensities exhibited by patients who seek voluntary admission

▶ The patient may be confined involuntarily in an appropriate facility for up to 72 hours without a temporary court order; however, the facility must begin court proceedings for involuntary commitment soon after confinement

▶ The court must immediately review an application for a temporary court order authorizing retention of the patient; if there is probable cause to believe that involuntary commitment is necessary, the court will issue the temporary order pending a final hearing

 • Probable cause means it's more probable than not that the patient will be involuntarily committed after the final hearing

 • At this point, the patient still hasn't been involuntarily committed

 • If the court finds that probable cause doesn't exist, the patient must be discharged

▶ If probable cause is found to exist, a final hearing must be conducted within 20 days of admission; the patient has the right to attend the final hearing and must be represented by counsel

▶ The court will authorize involuntary commitment if it finds clear and convincing evidence (beyond a reasonable doubt) of the need; if clear and convincing evidence doesn't exist, the patient must be discharged

▶ Periodic court review and hearings for all involuntarily committed patients must be conducted 3, 9, and 12 months from the date of the first hearing and annually thereafter

▶ If a psychiatric facility determines that a patient no longer needs involuntary commitment, the patient can be discharged pursuant to a statutorily required discharge plan

◆ The statutory procedures required for voluntary admission and involuntary commitment were designed to protect a person's right to liberty, due process, and equal protection under the law

■ Seclusion or restraint of a psychiatric patient may be needed under certain circumstances

◆ Seclusion and restraint are interventions used to protect a psychiatric patient from the likelihood of injury to self or others; such interventions shouldn't be used for staff convenience or to punish or coerce patients

▶ Restraint is usually accomplished through the application of such devices as cloth or leather wrist and ankle restraints

▶ Seclusion is usually accomplished by isolating a patient in a locked room

◆ Numerous legal implications surround a determination to restrict a psychiatric patient

▶ The doctrine of least restrictive treatment requires the use of restrictive measures only if necessary and only to the extent required to ensure the safety of the patient and others; therefore, if a vest is adequate to restrain a patient, a four-point restraint shouldn't be used

▶ Seclusion or restraint must be used for the minimum amount of time necessary and only when less restrictive measures have proved ineffective; all earlier less restrictive measures attempted must be documented

▶ If a patient is competent, informed consent must be obtained before seclusion or restraints are used

▶ If a patient is incompetent or a minor, consent must be obtained from the patient's legal guardian or parent; in an emergency, the requirement to obtain informed consent doesn't apply

▶ If a patient suddenly becomes violent and is in imminent danger of self-harm or causing harm to others, action can be taken without the patient's consent

▶ Many state laws limit the use of seclusion and restraint to occasions when the patient has attempted injury to self or others or has caused significant property damage

▶ Many facilities have specific policies and procedures for using seclusion and restraint

▶ Nurses should be thoroughly familiar with their state's statutes and with their facility's policies and procedures

▶ Failure to use restrictive measures when indicated could expose a nurse to claims for injury to the patient or a third party, such as another patient or staff member

◆ When seclusion or restraints have been implemented, additional legal issues arise

▶ An inappropriate decision to restrain or isolate a patient could expose a nurse to allegations of assault, battery, and false imprisonment; explicit documentation of the patient's behavior, the reason for the restriction, and justification for the type of restriction used are necessary

▶ Patients who are restrained must be afforded maximum freedom of movement while assuring the physical safety of themselves and others

▶ Continual observation of the secluded or restrained patient is vitally important, and the extent of the observation should be documented

▶ Any time a patient is restrained, that patient is vulnerable to harm due to the inability to defend himself or herself; the restrained patient must be kept secluded and safe from other patients during the time of the restraint

▶ State statutes and health facility policies and procedures address the requirements for a physician's order, its renewal, the length of time a patient may remain secluded or restrained, the need for observation, and the maintenance of the patient's hygiene

▶ The psychiatric and mental health nurse must be familiar with these requirements and adhere to them

❖ Assault and battery

- Assault is an attempt or threat to unlawfully touch or injure another person; apprehension resulting from the potential contact is what gives rise to claims of assault
- Battery is the unlawful and intentional touching of another
- Assault and battery are intentional torts
- Claims of assault or battery can arise in the psychiatric setting under several circumstances
    - ◆ The patient assaults or batters another patient, a staff member, or a third party
    - ◆ The patient assaults or batters the nurse
    - ◆ A staff member assaults or batters a patient or is accused of having done so
- The psychiatric and mental health nurse must attempt to prevent these situations from happening and know the steps to take if an assault or battery situation arises
    - ◆ Professional literature has identified patient profiles and situations that lead to assault and battery by patients
        - ▶ The nurse should evaluate each patient for the potential to engage in assault and battery
            - • Has the patient previously assaulted or battered anyone?
            - • Is the patient taking a medication, such as fluoxetine (Prozac), that is associated with patient violence?
            - • Does the patient have a history of difficulty with authority?

▶ After identifying a patient's predisposition to assault and battery, the nurse should institute close observation and preventive interventions and document these measures in the patient's medical record

▶ Situations that may precipitate patient violence include:
  • Involuntary confinement
  • Invasion of a patient's personal space
  • Limiting a patient's behavior
  • Staff attitude toward a patient

▶ Nurses should intervene to help a patient cope with these events and conduct staff teaching on appropriate attitudes

▶ If a nurse fails to act reasonably to prevent a patient from assaulting or battering a third party, the nurse could be found liable for the third party's injuries

◆ Staff abuse of patients does occur; a psychiatric and mental health nurse who has reason to believe that a staff member is abusing a patient should report the suspicion to a supervisor or begin an appropriate investigation

◆ Each health care facility should have policies and procedures that address these situations

◆ Patients have brought claims of assault and battery against psychiatric and mental health nurses for implementing seclusion and restraint and for administering treatments, including forced medication, without the patient's consent

❖ Patient rights

■ Psychiatric patients are entitled to the same rights that other patients enjoy

◆ A psychiatric patient may not be deprived of any constitutional or common law right simply because of receiving psychiatric treatment

◆ In some instances, psychiatric patients are granted special legal protection because of their vulnerable status

■ Basic patient rights include:
  ◆ The right to receive quality health care
  ◆ The right to informed consent and informed refusal
  ◆ The right to privacy
  ◆ The right to have medical information treated in a confidential manner
  ◆ The right to obtain a copy of one's medical records, unless medically inadvisable
  ◆ The right to receive treatment without discrimination because of race, age, sex, religion, ethnicity, or inability to pay
  ◆ The right to maintain one's dignity

■ Many state laws contain specific requirements to protect the rights of psychiatric patients

♦ A psychiatric patient's rights are violated if the patient is:
  ▶ Presumed to be incompetent merely because of being mentally ill
  ▶ Given unnecessary or excessive medication as a punishment, for the convenience of staff, or as a substitute for treatment
  ▶ Subjected to experimental treatment, electroconvulsive treatment, psychosurgery, or sterilization without informed consent or judicial authorization
    • A competent patient must be given the right to consult an attorney or anyone else and must give express written consent for such treatment
    • If the patient is incompetent, a court hearing must be held with the patient present and represented by counsel, and the treatment must be judicially authorized before it can be rendered
  ▶ Restrained or secluded unless such restraint or seclusion is legally permitted
  ▶ Subjected to corporal punishment
♦ Specific psychiatric patient rights include:
  ▶ The right to the least restrictive treatment
  ▶ The right to have one's own clothing, limited personal possessions, and a place to store them
  ▶ The right to receive visitors, make phone calls, and write letters
♦ Many state laws require that a psychiatric patient's rights be posted, given, or recited to the patient on admission or shortly thereafter
■ Psychiatric patients have the right to privileged communication and confidentiality
  ♦ Communications between a psychiatric patient and the health care provider are legally protected as privileged communications by state law; this means that information about the patient must be kept confidential unless the privilege is waived by the patient or some exception to nondisclosure exists
    ▶ Privileged communication statutes differ from state to state
    ▶ Most states don't specifically include nurses in the category of health care providers subject to a privileged communication statute
    ▶ If information disclosed to the nurse is necessary for treatment of the patient, the information may be considered privileged; however, some courts will require a nurse to disclose confidential information if a specific statutory privilege for nurse-patient communication doesn't exist
  ♦ Nurses are required to maintain a patient's right to confidentiality, with some exceptions
    ▶ A nurse is required to report acts of child abuse; if a psychiatric patient admits to committing such acts, the nurse must disclose this information to the appropriate authorities
    ▶ If a psychiatric patient threatens to harm someone, the nurse may have the duty to warn the intended victim or take some other action to make the threat known to a supervisor or civil authority

◆ Because of the sensitive nature of the information contained in a psychiatric patient's records, the federal government and some states have enacted legislation that provides special confidentiality protection to patients receiving drug and alcohol abuse treatment and psychological treatment

◆ If a nurse discloses confidential information about the patient without the patient's consent, a claim of invasion of privacy or breach of confidentiality may ensue

❖ Documentation of care

■ Although mental health records are primarily maintained to foster communication among health care providers and thereby facilitate delivery of appropriate care, they also serve certain legal purposes

◆ Mental health records are used as evidence in competency hearings and involuntary commitment hearings

◆ They are also used as evidence in lawsuits when a patient claims a health care provider has acted negligently or committed an intentional tort

◆ Although mental health records are considered confidential, their contents may be disclosed during any legal proceeding as long as the information is reasonably related to the matter undergoing judicial review

■ A patient's mental health records, whether manual or computerized, must be properly protected to prevent access by unauthorized individuals

◆ Access to a patient's mental health records must be limited to those health care providers who are involved in treating the patient

◆ A patient's mental health records may be reviewed for the purposes of peer review, quality assurance, audits, and research; however, the confidentiality of the information gathered must be protected, and any report generated as a result of such reviews must not directly or indirectly identify the patient

◆ A patient's mental health records or information derived from them should never be released to third parties, such as insurance companies, without the patient's written authorization

■ Documentation appearing in the medical record should be objective, concise, and thorough; only pertinent information should be charted

◆ Because the patient has the legal right of access to treatment records, the psychiatric and mental health nurse should chart as if the patient were reading the record

◆ Documentation should reflect treatment rendered in accordance with prevailing standards of nursing care

▶ If the nurse's actions are subsequently questioned (for example, in a lawsuit), the nurse will be able to demonstrate that the correct standard of care was met

▶ Courts generally assume that treatment wasn't given unless it's documented in the patient's record

▶ If a nurse testifies that certain treatment was rendered but it doesn't appear in the record, the nurse may not be believed, especially if the testimony is about an incident that occurred several years before the testimony

◆ A patient's mental health record should never be altered to conceal a negligent act; a patient's injury or an incorrect treatment should be charted without concluding who was at fault

❖ Child protection (or protective) laws

■ The psychiatric nurse must be alert for any signs and symptoms of child abuse and report any suspected abuse to the appropriate authorities

■ Many states have laws that say any person who has reason to believe that a child is being abused, neglected or abandoned must report this to Child Protection Services or to the police within 24 hours; failure to report suspected abuse, neglect or abandonment is a misdemeanor (subject to penalties) in some states

■ Some state laws indicate that only professionals, such as physicians, registered nurses, dentists, social workers, and mental health professionals are required to report suspected child abuse

■ Potential victims must be warned of or protected from possible harm; if a psychiatric patient has indicated actual abuse or thoughts of abuse of a child, this must be reported to Child Protection Services; the patient should remain hospitalized or kept from the child until the patient's condition has stabilized and an investigation by Child Protection Services has been completed

Review questions

1. Four elements of nursing negligence are present in an unintentional tort; the nurse owes the patient a duty of care, the nurse breaches the duty of care, the patient suffers damages, and:

○ **A.** the nurse intentionally harms the patient.

○ **B.** the nurse's breach of duty causes the patient's damages.

○ **C.** the nurse breaches the patient's confidentiality.

○ **D.** the nurse doesn't obtain informed consent.

Correct answer: B The fourth element of an unintentional tort is that the nurse's breach of duty caused the damage claimed by the patient. Intentional harm, breach of confidentiality, and failure to obtain informed consent are intentional torts, in which an intent to commit the act is present.

2. Battery or assault charges can result from which of the following situations?

    ○ **A.** Restraining a patient who is attempting to harm himself

    ○ **B.** Secluding an escalating patient when other de-escalating measures have failed

    ○ **C.** A patient harming a nurse or staff member

    ○ **D.** Breach of confidentiality by the nurse

Correct answer: C   Claims of assault or battery can arise in the psychiatric setting if the patient harms a nurse or staff member. Restraining a patient who is attempting to harm himself isn't considered battery if other measures have been tried unsuccessfully and such restrictive measures are used only to the extent required to ensure the safety of the patient and others. Seclusion of an escalating patient is justified when other measures have proven ineffective. Breach of confidentiality isn't considered battery.

3. The best way to handle an escalating patient is to:

    ○ **A.** assess the patient's medication history.

    ○ **B.** seclude the patient.

    ○ **C.** assess for the patient's potential for violence.

    ○ **D.** intervene early to de-escalate the situation.

Correct answer: D   Early intervention to de-escalate the situation can prevent the need for seclusion or restraints. Medication history is important but not helpful in the immediate situation. Assessment for violence is important but not necessarily helpful in de-escalating the patient.

4. A restrained patient is usually kept in locked seclusion for which of the following reasons?

    ○ **A.** The silence available in locked seclusion will help calm the patient.

    ○ **B.** The patient must be protected from others while restrained.

    ○ **C.** Seclusion will lessen the need for patient observation while restrained.

    ○ **D.** Seclusion rooms are usually closer to the nurses' station.

Correct answer: B   Seclusion is an intervention used to protect a psychiatric patient from the likelihood of injury to self or others. Any patient in seclusion requires additional, not less, observation. A patient isn't secluded in order to be closer to the nurse's station. Locked seclusion isn't required in order for the patient to be in a quiet environment.

Anxiety disorders

❖ Overview
- Anxiety is a subjective feeling of vague apprehension that a person experiences in response to stress
- Anxiety serves two primary purposes
  - ◆ It alerts the person to an actual or impending danger
  - ◆ It prepares the person to take defensive action (fight or flight)
- Some forms of anxiety are normal; other forms may signal a medical or psychological problem or a primary disorder
- Peplau classified anxiety by its intensity: mild, moderate, severe, or panic (see *Levels of anxiety*, page 82)
- More severe manifestations of anxiety can be dysfunctional, presenting in various syndromes characterized as anxiety disorders
- The syndromes are marked by an underlying anxiety that the person desperately tries to control
- The psychiatric and mental health nurse can detect anxious behavior in a patient by observing for certain physiologic, cognitive, and social-emotional responses (see *Responses to anxiety*, page 83)

❖ Theoretical perspectives
- Biological theory
  - ◆ Anxiety results from a biochemical imbalance between the norepinephrine system and other transmitter systems such as serotonin in the brain
  - ◆ Researchers are investigating the relationship between gamma-aminobutyric acid (GABA), the brain's main inhibitory transmitter system, and anxiety disorders
- Psychodynamic theory
  - ◆ Anxiety results from unresolved developmental conflicts (see chapter 3, Human development)
  - ◆ The ego erects defense mechanisms to protect itself from potentially overwhelming anxiety
- Interpersonal theory
  - ◆ Behavior is designed to attain security and satisfaction
  - ◆ Anxiety results when expectations or needs aren't met in interpersonal relationships

Levels of anxiety

Peplau classified anxiety according to its level of intensity: mild, moderate, severe, or panic. This chart presents the major characteristics of each anxiety level, along with appropriate nursing interventions.

Anxiety level	Characteristics	Nursing interventions
Mild	• Alertness • Optimum ability to solve problems and make independent decisions • Enhanced learning	• Support optimal functioning of the patient.
Moderate	• Hyperalertness and vigilance • Impaired problem-solving ability (assistance needed) • Selective inattention • Complaints of feeling "uptight"	• Assist the patient in talking through the experience and labeling accompanying feelings. • Show the connections between details. • Encourage the patient to use appropriate relaxation exercises.
Severe	• Narrowed patient focus • Severely impaired problem-solving skills • Inability to grasp meaning of communications, engage in self-directed activity, or make decisions • Numerous physiologic complaints • Dependence on others, demands for attention	• Provide the patient with structure and direction. • Remain with the patient and provide constant attention until anxiety diminishes to a moderate level. • Administer medication as needed.
Panic	• Complete inability to solve problems • Possible feelings of suffocation or loss of contact with reality • Inability to recognize familiar people, objects, or situations, even when identified by someone else • Erratic behavior	• Establish a simple, nonstimulating, structured environment. • Remain with the patient at all times. • Speak in quiet tones, and use touch cautiously. • Engage the patient in large-muscle or structured activity that doesn't require the ability to concentrate or solve problems.

■ Behavioral theory
◆ Anxiety is a learned response to stress
◆ Anxiety can be effectively reduced by using various behavioral techniques

❖ **Generalized anxiety disorder (GAD)**
■ Characteristics
◆ Excessive or unrealistic worry or apprehension about several aspects of life
◆ Inordinate amount of energy expended on controlling anxious feelings
■ Criteria for medical diagnosis (see the diagnostic criteria for GAD, page 84)
■ Selected nursing diagnoses
◆ Anxiety related to feeling of helplessness

Responses to anxiety

Individuals respond to anxiety in various ways. Some of these responses are normal; others may signal a serious health problem. A patient with an anxiety disorder, for example, typically exhibits many of the physical, cognitive, and social-emotional responses to anxiety listed below. These signs and symptoms can assist the nurse in formulating nursing diagnoses appropriate for the patient's condition.

Responses	Nursing diagnoses
Physical	
• Restlessness	• Fatigue
• Tremulousness	• Acute pain
• Increased pulse and respirations	• Disturbed sensory perception (visual)
• Elevated blood pressure	• Disturbed sleep pattern
• Tightness in chest, neck, or back	• Impaired urinary elimination
• Breathing difficulty	• Ineffective breathing pattern
• Perspiration	• Constipation
• Insomnia	• Diarrhea
• Headache	
• Nausea	
• Dizziness	
• Fatigue	
• Urinary urgency, frequency, or both	
• Constipation or diarrhea	
Cognitive	
• Inattentiveness, distractibility	• Impaired verbal communication
• Poor concentration	• Disturbed thought processes
• Forgetfulness	
• Blocking of thoughts	
• Rumination	
• Preoccupation such as with body functions	
• Decreased ability to solve problems	
Social-emotional	
• Vague feeling of discomfort	• Anxiety
• Apprehension	• Fear
• Worry	• Impaired parenting
• Expectation of danger	• Ineffective role performance
• Irritability	• Social isolation
• Lack of self-confidence	• Spiritual distress
• Tendency to cry easily	• Risk for self-directed violence
• Social withdrawal	• Imbalanced nutrition: Less than body requirements
• Inappropriate responses to a social situation	• Ineffective sexuality patterns

◆ Fatigue related to insomnia
◆ Disturbed sleep pattern related to inability to relax
◆ Ineffective health maintenance related to inattention to activities of daily living (ADLs)

(Text continues on page 87.)

Diagnostic criteria for anxiety disorders

Here are *DSM-IV-TR* diagnostic criteria for the anxiety disorders discussed in this chapter.

Generalized anxiety disorder

A. The person experiences excessive anxiety and worry (apprehensive expectation) more days than not for at least 6 months about a number of events or activities (such as work or school performance).

B. The person finds it difficult to control the worry.

C. The anxiety and worry are associated with three or more of the following six symptoms (with at least some symptoms present for more days than not for the past 6 months). *Note:* Only one symptom is required in children.
   1. Restlessness or a feeling of being keyed up or on edge
   2. Being easily fatigued
   3. Difficulty concentrating or mind going blank
   4. Irritability
   5. Muscle tension
   6. Sleep disturbance (difficulty falling or staying asleep or restless, unsatisfying sleep)

D. The focus of the anxiety and worry is not confined to features of an Axis I disorder; for example, the anxiety or worry is not about having a panic attack (as in panic disorder), being embarrassed in public (as in social phobia), being contaminated (as in obsessive-compulsive disorder), being away from home or close relatives (as in separation anxiety disorder), gaining weight (as in anorexia nervosa), having multiple physical complaints (as in somatization disorder), or having a serious illness (as in hypochondriasis), and the anxiety and worry do not occur exclusively during posttraumatic stress disorder.

E. The anxiety, worry, or physical symptoms cause clinically significant distress or impairment in social, occupational, or other important areas of functioning.

F. The disturbance is not due to the direct physiologic effects of a substance (such as a drug of abuse or a medication) or of a general medical condition (such as hyperthyroidism) and does not occur exclusively during a mood disorder, a psychotic disorder, or a pervasive developmental disorder.

Panic disorder without agoraphobia

A. The person experiences recurrent unexpected panic attacks, at least one of which has been followed by 1 month or more of at least one of the following:
   1. Persistent concern about having additional attacks
   2. Worry about the implications of the attack or its consequences (losing control, having a heart attack, "going crazy")
   3. A significant change in behavior related to the attacks

B. Absence of agoraphobia

C. The panic attacks are not due to the direct physiologic effects of a substance (such as a drug of abuse or a medication) or a general medical condition (such as hyperthyroidism).

D. The panic attacks are not better accounted for by another mental disorder, such as social phobia (for example, occurring on exposure to feared social situations), specific phobia (on exposure to a specific phobic situation), obsessive-compulsive disorder (on exposure to dirt in someone with an obsession about contamination), posttraumatic stress disorder (in response to stimuli associated with a severe stressor), or separation anxiety disorder (in response to being away from home or close relatives).

Panic disorder with agoraphobia

A. The person experiences recurrent unexpected panic attacks, at least one of which has been followed by 1 month or more of at least one or more of the following:
   1. Persistent concern about having additional attacks
   2. Worry about the implications of the attack or its consequences (losing control, having a heart attack, "going crazy")
   3. A significant change in behavior related to the attacks

B. Presence of agoraphobia

C. The panic attacks are not due to the direct physiologic effects of a substance (such as a drug of abuse or a medication) or a general medical condition (such as hyperthyroidism).

D. The panic attacks are not better accounted for by another mental disorder, such as social phobia (for example,

Diagnostic criteria for anxiety disorders *(continued)*

occurring on exposure to feared social situations), specific phobia (on exposure to a specific phobic situation), obsessive-compulsive disorder (on exposure to dirt in someone with an obsession about contamination), post-traumatic stress disorder (in response to stimuli associated with a severe stressor), or separation anxiety disorder (in response to being away from home or close relatives).

Obsessive-compulsive disorder

A. The person experiences either obsessions or compulsions.
   1. *Obsessions* are recurrent and persistent thoughts, impulses, or images that are experienced, at some time during the disturbance, as intrusive and inappropriate and that cause marked anxiety or distress.
      a. The thoughts, impulses, or images are not simply excessive worries about real-life problems.
      b. The person attempts to ignore or suppress such thoughts, impulses, or images or to neutralize them with some other thought or action.
      c. The person recognizes that the obsessional thoughts, impulses, or images are a product of his or her own mind (not imposed from without as in thought insertion).
   2. *Compulsions* are repetitive behaviors (such as hand washing, ordering, checking) or mental acts (praying, counting, repeating words silently) that the person feels driven to perform in response to an obsession or according to rules that must be applied rigidly.
      a. The behaviors or mental acts are aimed at preventing or reducing distress or preventing some dreaded event or situation.
      b. These behaviors or mental acts either are not connected in a realistic way with what they are designed to neutralize or prevent or are clearly excessive.
B. At some point during the course of the disorder, the person has recognized that the obsessions or compulsions are excessive or unreasonable. *Note:* This does not apply to children.
C. The obsessions or compulsions cause marked distress, are time-consuming (take more than 1 hour per day), or significantly interfere with the person's normal routine, occupational or academic functioning, or usual social activities or relationships.
D. If another Axis I disorder is present, the content of the obsessions or compulsions is not restricted to it (for example, preoccupation with food in the presence of an eating disorder; hair pulling in the presence of trichotillomania; concern with appearance in the presence of body dysmorphic disorder; preoccupation with drugs in the presence of a substance use disorder; preoccupation with having a serious illness in the presence of hypochondriasis; preoccupation with sexual urges or fantasies in the presence of a paraphilia; or guilty ruminations in the presence of major depressive disorder).
E. The disturbance is not due to the direct physiologic effects of a substance (such as a drug of abuse or a medication) or of a general medical condition.
   Specify **with poor insight** if, for most of the time during the current episode, the person does not recognize that the obsessions and compulsions are excessive or unreasonable.

Specific phobia

A. The person experiences marked and persistent fear that is excessive or unreasonable, cued by the presence or anticipation of a specific object or situation (flying, heights, animals, receiving an injection, seeing blood).
B. Exposure to the phobic stimulus almost invariably provokes an immediate anxiety response, which may take the form of a situationally bound or situationally predisposed panic attack. *Note:* In children, the anxiety may be expressed by crying, tantrums, freezing, or clinging.
C. The person recognizes that the fear is excessive or unreasonable. *Note:* In children, this feature may be absent.
D. The phobic situation is avoided or else is endured with intense anxiety or distress.
E. The avoidance, anxious anticipation, or distress in the feared situation interferes significantly with the person's normal routine, occupational or academic functioning, or social activities or relationships, or there is marked distress about having the phobia.
F. In individuals under age 18, the duration is at least 6 months.
G. The anxiety, panic attack, or phobic avoidance associated with the specific object or situation is not better accounted for by another mental disorder, such as obsessive-compulsive disorder (such as fear of dirt in someone with an obsession about contamination), posttraumatic stress disorder (avoidance of stimuli associated with a severe stressor), separation anxiety disorder (avoidance of school), social phobia (avoidance of social situations

(continued)

Diagnostic criteria for anxiety disorders *(continued)*

because of fear of embarrassment), panic disorder with agoraphobia, or agoraphobia without history of panic disorder.

Specify type:
   Animal type
   Natural environment type (for example, heights, storms, water)
   Blood-injection-injury type (this type is highly familial and is commonly characterized by a strong vasovagal response)
   Situational type (for example, being on bridges or in tunnels, airplanes, cars, elevators, or other enclosed places
   Other type (for example, fear of choking, vomiting, open space, or contracting an illness; in children, fear of loud sounds or costumed characters)

Posttraumatic stress disorder

A. The person has been exposed to a traumatic event in which both of the following were present:
   1. The person experienced, witnessed, or was confronted with an event that involved actual or threatened death or serious injury or a threat to the physical integrity of self or others.
   2. The person's response involved intense fear, helplessness, or horror. *Note:* In children, this may be expressed instead by disorganized or agitated behavior.
B. The traumatic event is persistently reexperienced in one (or more) of the following ways:
   1. Recurrent and intrusive distressing recollections of the event, including images, thoughts, or perceptions. *Note:* In young children, repetitive play may occur in which themes or aspects of the trauma are expressed.
   2. Recurrent distressing dreams of the event. *Note:* In children, there may be frightening dreams without recognizable content.
   3. Acting or feeling as if the traumatic event were recurring (includes a sense of reliving the experience, illusions, hallucinations, and dissociative flashback episodes, including those that occur on awakening or when intoxicated). *Note:* In young children, trauma-specific reenactment may occur.
   4. Intense psychological distress at exposure to internal or external cues that symbolize or resemble an aspect of the traumatic event
   5. Physiologic reactivity on exposure to internal or external cues that symbolize or resemble an aspect of the traumatic event
C. The person persistently avoids stimuli associated with the trauma and numbing of general responsiveness (not present before the trauma), as indicated by three or more of the following:
   1. Efforts to avoid thoughts, feelings, or conversations associated with the trauma
   2. Efforts to avoid activities, places, or people that arouse recollections of the trauma
   3. Inability to recall an important aspect of the trauma
   4. Markedly diminished interest or participation in significant activities
   5. Feeling of detachment or estrangement from others
   6. Restricted range of affect (such as an inability to have loving feelings)
   7. Sense of foreshortened future (such as not expecting to have a career, marriage, children, or a normal life span)
D. The person experiences persistent symptoms of increased arousal (not present before the trauma) as indicated by two (or more) of the following:
   1. Difficulty falling or staying asleep
   2. Irritability or outbursts of anger
   3. Difficulty concentrating
   4. Hypervigilance
   5. Exaggerated startle response
E. Duration of the disturbance (symptoms in criteria B, C, and D) is more than 1 month.
F. The disturbance causes clinically significant distress or impairment in social, occupational, or other important areas of functioning.
   Specify **acute** if duration of symptoms is less than 3 months; **chronic** if 3 months or more. *Specify* **with delayed onset** if onset of symptoms is at least 6 months after the stressor.

Adapted from *Diagnostic and Statistical Manual of Mental Disorders*, 4th ed., text revision. Washington, D.C.: American Psychiatric Association, 2000, with permission of the publisher.

◆ Impaired social interaction related to withdrawal from social contacts
■ Treatment
  ◆ Relaxation training (breathing exercises, progressive muscle relaxation, guided imagery)
  ◆ Benzodiazepine therapy (early phase of treatment, optional)
  ◆ Selective serotonin reuptake inhibitors or serotonin and norepinephrine reuptake inhibitors and buspirone (BuSpar)
  ◆ Psychotherapy
  ◆ Education
■ General nursing interventions
  ◆ Assist the patient in identifying events that tend to increase anxiety and events during which the patient experiences relative internal calm
  ◆ Engage the patient in anticipatory planning
  ◆ Teach the patient about relaxation techniques, and practice them with the patient
  ◆ Help the patient work on one problem at a time
  ◆ Accompany the patient to activities that the patient is too anxious to attend alone
  ◆ Teach the patient about cognitive interventions such as positive self-talk training
  ◆ Instruct the patient in the use of sensory interventions, such as music therapy or aroma therapy

❖ **Panic disorder**
  ■ Characteristics
    ◆ Episodes of extreme panic that can last from a few minutes to a few hours
    ◆ Relatively anxiety-free periods between attacks of panic-level anxiety (unlike with GAD)
    ◆ Fear of future attacks because the episodes are unpredictable and the patient feels out of control during them
    ◆ Attempts by the patient to impose severe limitations on lifestyle in order to stave off future attacks
    ◆ Possible development of phobias as the patient tries to avoid anything associated with panic attacks
  ■ Criteria for medical diagnosis (see the diagnostic criteria for panic disorder, pages 84 and 85)
  ■ Selected nursing diagnoses
    ◆ Anxiety related to extreme, unrealistic fear
    ◆ Risk for injury related to feeling of terror
    ◆ Ineffective coping related to apprehension and helplessness
    ◆ Impaired social interaction related to inability to differentiate harmful situations from safe ones
  ■ Treatment
    ◆ Benzodiazepine (such as alprazolam [Xanax])

◆ Antidepressants (such as sertraline [Zoloft] or paroxetine [Paxil])
◆ Relaxation techniques
◆ Aerobic exercise (only after careful evaluation; some patients have experienced panic attacks from lactic acid buildup after exercise)
■ General nursing interventions
◆ Remain with the patient during a panic attack
◆ Provide for safety needs to counter the patient's impaired perception
◆ Administer medication as needed
◆ Help the patient find a pattern to the attacks (for example, after vigorous exercise, during certain times of the day, at specific places or events)

❖ Obsessive-compulsive disorder
■ Characteristics
◆ Recurrent and persistent thoughts, images, or impulses (obsessions) that the patient doesn't want but can't ignore
◆ Irrational, repetitive, ritualistic behaviors (compulsions) that the patient uses in attempts to control the anxiety resulting from obsessions
◆ Inability to control the thoughts and behaviors, despite recognition by the patient of their absurdity and intensity
◆ Marked interference with normal daily routines, consuming hours of the patient's day
◆ Possible benefits (secondary gains) that the patient experiences, thereby perpetuating the obsessive-compulsive behavior
■ Criteria for medical diagnosis (see the diagnostic criteria for obsessive-compulsive disorder, page 85)
■ Selected nursing diagnoses
◆ Anxiety related to feelings that are unacceptable to the patient
◆ Risk for self-directed violence related to compulsive behaviors such as mutilation
◆ Risk for other-directed violence related to hostility or aggression
◆ Chronic low self-esteem related to unwanted obsessive thoughts
◆ Ineffective health maintenance related to disruptions in carrying out ADLs
◆ Impaired verbal communication related to reduced ability to express unwanted feelings
■ Treatment
◆ Behavioral techniques
▶ Desensitization, or graded exposure (having the patient gradually engage in anxiety-provoking activities or situations)
▶ Modeling of desired behavior (showing the patient how to respond to bothersome stimuli)
▶ Response delay (having the patient wait for increasingly longer intervals before engaging in ritualistic behaviors)

▶ Cognitive therapy such as thought stopping (having the patient willfully interrupt unwanted, anxiety-producing thoughts by engaging in a competing activity or by yelling "stop")
   ◆ Antidepressants (such as paroxetine [Paxil] or fluvoxamine [Luvox])
   ◆ Nonreinforcement of secondary gains
■ General nursing interventions
   ◆ Provide time for the patient to carry out rituals
   ◆ Don't interrupt a ritual after it has started; to do so could result in panic-level anxiety
   ◆ Assist the patient with self-care as needed
   ◆ Have the patient keep a journal about the events surrounding obsessive-compulsive behaviors
   ◆ Provide education

❖ **Specific phobia**
   ■ Characteristics
      ◆ Intense and unrealistic fear of an object, person, or event
      ◆ Willingness of the patient to do anything to avoid the phobic object, person, or event, regardless of the consequences
      ◆ Inability of the patient to overcome the fear, despite recognition by the patient that the fear is absurd
      ◆ Extreme anxiety on encountering the phobic object, person, or event
   ■ Criteria for medical diagnosis (see the diagnostic criteria for specific phobia, pages 85 and 86)
   ■ Selected nursing diagnoses
      ◆ Fear related to an irrational feeling toward something harmless
      ◆ Powerlessness related to an inability to control the fear
      ◆ Social isolation related to self-protected avoidance
   ■ Treatment
      ◆ Behavioral techniques
         ▶ Social-skills training, especially effective in ameliorating social phobia (fear and avoidance of a particular social situation)
         ▶ Desensitization, effective in ameliorating simple phobia and agoraphobia (fear and avoidance of public places)
      ◆ Benzodiazepine therapy (may be used to manage panic attacks, especially in agoraphobia)
   ■ General nursing interventions
      ◆ Never force the patient to contact the phobic object; such contact may precipitate a panic attack
      ◆ Instruct the patient in the behavioral techniques prescribed by the treatment team
      ◆ Reassure the patient that he won't be forced to confront the phobic situation
      ◆ Initially, adjust the environment to accommodate the patient's phobia; as treatment progresses, adjustment won't be necessary

❖ Posttraumatic stress disorder (PTSD)

- ■ Characteristics
  - ◆ Grieving-like behaviors that result from a major and severe trauma, such as rape, assault, accident, fire, war, or natural disaster
  - ◆ Extreme anxiety or fear and a sense of powerlessness or helplessness
  - ◆ Varying onset and intensity of symptoms
    - ▶ Acute PTSD: less than 3 months after the event
    - ▶ Chronic PTSD: 3 months or more after the event
    - ▶ Delayed PTSD: at least 6 months after the event
  - ◆ Extreme anxiety generated by reexperiencing the event (may lead to bouts of depression, substance abuse, or suicide attempts)
- ■ Criteria for medical diagnosis (see the diagnostic criteria for PTSD, page 86)
- ■ Selected nursing diagnoses
  - ◆ Posttrauma syndrome related to the traumatic experience
  - ◆ Risk for self-directed violence related to anger and self-blame over the event
  - ◆ Disturbed sleep pattern related to persistent dreams about the event
  - ◆ Anxiety related to feelings of insecurity and being unsafe
- ■ Treatment
  - ◆ Psychotherapy (directed toward helping the patient achieve cognitive mastery over the traumatic situation)
  - ◆ Benzodiazepine therapy (may be prescribed to manage uncontrollable anxiety)
  - ◆ Antidepressant therapy
- ■ General nursing interventions
  - ◆ Encourage the patient to recall the traumatic event; remain nonjudgmental and accept what the patient is saying
  - ◆ Provide a secure environment for the patient to promote a sense of safety
  - ◆ Remain with the patient, especially one who's extremely anxious; reexperiencing the traumatic event can trigger severe or panic anxiety
  - ◆ Institute suicide precautions if the patient manifests suicidal tendencies
  - ◆ Facilitate grieving by encouraging the patient to express emotions generated from the event
  - ◆ Teach the patient and family about posttraumatic behavior, and refer them to support groups for additional help

Clinical situation

You're employed in a community mental health center. One of your new patients is Paul Smith, a 38-year-old accountant who says that he worries excessively about making mistakes. In fact, he's so preoccupied with doing things correctly that he has been unable to function efficiently at work.

At home, Paul directs his energies toward making sure the family's finances are in order and checking up on the activities of his wife and children. He also worries about how neighbors and friends perceive him.

Paul tells you that he's exhausted from inadequate sleep and that he has experienced heartburn almost daily for the past several weeks. He describes himself as a worrywart, saying that he's always been a nervous person who's easily upset when unforeseen things happen. He confesses that the quality of his life is poor and that he's willing to do whatever it takes to stop worrying so much.

Assessment (nursing behaviors and rationales)

1. Perform a health assessment, especially inquiring about any changes in Paul's appetite, sleeping, digestion, elimination, and cardiac functioning. *Anxiety causes changes in physiologic processes. Any deterioration in physical health will need attention, and any physiologic cause for physical manifestations must be ruled out.*

2. Conduct a psychosocial assessment, especially inquiring about changes in Paul's coping patterns, social supports, financial status, occupational stressors, and interactional patterns. *A psychosocial assessment will assist in determining the severity of impairment resulting from anxiety and factors associated with anxiety.*

3. Assess Paul's perception of the current situation. *When planning and delivering appropriate care, the nurse must consider the patient's perceptions. Until the nurse can determine how the patient views the current situation, generating a care plan specific to this patient will be impossible.*

4. Assess Paul's ability to solve problems. *Such an assessment will help the nurse determine the patient's anxiety level. A particularly anxious patient won't be able to solve problems independently.*

Nursing diagnoses

- Anxiety related to the patient's need to be perfect
- Fatigue related to the patient's inability to sleep restfully at night and to feel relaxed during the day
- Ineffective role performance related to excessive worrying about doing everything well
- Acute pain related to gastric reflux

Planning and goals

- Paul Smith will learn to manage anxiety so that role performance is unaffected.
- He'll learn to relax during the day and to sleep more restfully at night.
- He'll no longer experience discomfort from gastric reflux.

Implementation (nursing behaviors and rationales)

1. Involve Paul in a physical and psychosocial assessment. *This activity not only provides valuable baseline data but also communicates concern about the pa-*

tient's well-being and the conviction that the patient is an active participant in his healing.

2. Have Paul identify his most pressing problems. *After the patient has completed this exercise, he's in a position to determine which problem to tackle first. As he begins to deal with problems, he'll feel empowered and, consequently, less anxious.*

3. Teach Paul how to engage in anticipatory planning rather than unproductive worrying. *Developing strategies in advance to manage potential problems will enhance the patient's self-control.*

4. Engage Paul in cognitive exercises (for example, "What if...?" or "What would be the worst possible thing that could happen?"). *Learning to use these cognitive techniques can help the patient avoid the trap of automatically becoming anxious when he feels stressed or unsure about a situation. Instead, he'll be able to develop a more objective perspective. When the patient learns to interrupt his automatic tendency to become anxious, he'll be better able to manage his life.*

5. Teach Paul relaxation techniques to use as soon as he becomes aware of feeling tense or nervous. *Like cognitive exercises, relaxation techniques will interrupt the patient's automatic tendency to become anxious and will enhance his ability to maintain a balanced body chemistry.*

Evaluation

- Paul Smith uses a series of cognitive exercises and relaxation techniques in the morning before arising and during the day when he becomes aware of feeling tense.
- Paul sleeps restfully at night and reports having abundant energy throughout the day.
- Paul no longer experiences gastric reflux.
- Paul reports that he no longer feels a constant need to check up on family members and that his productivity level at work has increased markedly.

Review questions

1. Which statement best explains the biological theory of anxiety?

○ **A.** A biochemical imbalance exists between the norepinephrine system and other transmitter systems in the brain.

○ **B.** Catecholamines are increased in the temporal lobe of the brain.

○ **C.** The GABA receptors in the limbic system are more sensitive to anxiety-producing biological effects.

○ **D.** Unresolved conflicts create psychological pain.

Correct answer: A Researchers think that an imbalance exists between norepinephrine and other transmitter systems within the brain. The role of catecholamines and GABA receptors remains under investigation. It's unknown how psychological pain is physically produced.

2. Which criterion differentiates panic disorder from GAD?

○ **A.** Periods of severe depression

○ **B.** Relatively anxiety-free periods between attacks

○ **C.** Risk of dependence on alcohol

○ **D.** Risk of dependence on benzodiazepines

Correct answer: B The patient with panic disorder is relatively anxiety-free for periods between attacks of panic-level anxiety, whereas the patient with GAD typically experiences anxiety more often than not over 6 months. Periods of severe depression and dependence on alcohol or benzodiazepines aren't characteristic of panic disorders but may indicate a more severe problem with anxiety or depression.

3. Which factor is most likely to cause disturbed sleep pattern in patients with PTSD?

○ **A.** Drinking alcohol at bedtime

○ **B.** Fear of being harmed while asleep

○ **C.** Adverse reactions to medications

○ **D.** Persistent dreams of the traumatic event

Correct answer: D Persistent dreams of the traumatic event result in sleep disorders. Drinking alcohol at bedtime and adverse reactions to medications aren't commonly associated with sleep disturbances. The patient doesn't usually fear being harmed while asleep.

4. Which of the following nursing interventions is most appropriate for a patient with obsessive-compulsive disorder?

○ **A.** Encouraging the patient to concentrate on and pay attention to unwanted thoughts

○ **B.** Giving antipsychotic medications as needed

○ **C.** Interrupting the patient's ritual to empower the patient in gaining control over the ritual

○ **D.** Providing time for the patient to carry out the ritual

Correct answer: D Allowing the patient time to carry out rituals is important because such behavior is aimed at preventing or reducing distress or preventing some dreaded event or situation from occurring. The ritual shouldn't be interrupted; otherwise, greater stress will occur. The patient should be encouraged to interrupt unwanted, anxiety-producing thoughts rather than focus on them. Antipsychotic medications are generally not necessary for a patient with obsessive-compulsive disorder.

Substance use disorders

CHAPTER 10

❖ Overview
- Addiction to psychoactive substances is a worldwide health problem
- The mind-altering substances most commonly abused to the point of addiction are alcohol, narcotics, hallucinogens, and stimulants
- Addiction (or chemical dependence, a term preferred by many health care professionals) is the end point of substance abuse; it's one of the most serious public health problems in the United States today
- The symptoms and maladaptive behaviors associated with chemical dependence are categorized according to the addictive substance (see *Diagnoses for substance use disorders*)
- Alcohol, by far the leading substance abused by Americans, is the principal focus of this section
- Other drug addictions are reviewed in the context of their common effects on the body and the usual treatment approaches (see *Diagnostic criteria for substance dependence*, page 96)

❖ Epidemiology of substance abuse
- Alcohol
  - About two-thirds of American adults consume alcohol; about 14% of them develop problems of dependence
  - Roughly one-third of all hospital admissions are related to alcohol abuse
  - The divorce rate for couples with an alcoholic spouse is seven times greater than that for other couples
  - Most high school students have tried alcohol by their senior year; about 6% of high school seniors consume alcohol daily
  - Approximately one-half of all traffic accidents are alcohol-related
- Drugs
  - Drug use is most prevalent among minority groups in metropolitan areas, but the problem crosses all racial, ethnic, socioeconomic, and geographic barriers
    - About 12% of all Americans have tried cocaine, which is used most commonly by young adults ages 18 to 25
    - About 3% of those ages 12 to 17 and 12% of those ages 18 to 25 have used lysergic acid diethylamide or phencyclidine
    - More than 50% of young adults have experimented with marijuana

Diagnoses for substance use disorders

Here is a list of the *DSM-IV-TR* diagnoses for substance use disorders.

Alcohol Dependence
Alcohol Abuse
Amphetamine Dependence
Amphetamine Abuse
Caffeine Intoxication
Cannabis Dependence
Cannabis Abuse
Cocaine Dependence
Cocaine Abuse
Hallucinogen Dependence
Hallucinogen Abuse
Inhalant Dependence

Inhalant Abuse
Nicotine Dependence
Opioid Dependence
Opioid Abuse
Phencyclidine Dependence
Phencyclidine Abuse
Sedative-Hypnotic or Anxiolytic Dependence
Sedative-Hypnotic or Anxiolytic Abuse
Polysubstance Dependence
Other (or Unknown) Substance Dependence
Other (or Unknown) Substance Abuse

Adapted from *Diagnostic and Statistical Manual of Mental Disorders*, 4th ed., text revision. Washington, D.C.: American Psychiatric Association, 2000 with permission of the publisher.

- ◆ Narcotics abusers typically abuse more than one drug
    - ▶ About 50% of abusers become chemically dependent
    - ▶ Drug abuse afflicts about 6% of those taking sedatives, 8% of those taking antianxiety agents, and 9% of those taking amphetamines
- ◆ One out of every two substance abusers meets the *DSM-IV-TR* diagnostic criteria for another mental illness, such as depression, schizophrenia, or borderline personality disorder

❖ Theoretical perspectives
- ■ Biological theory
    - ◆ Especially among those who abuse alcohol, a strong family history of abuse exists, suggesting a genetic link
    - ◆ Recent studies have shown evidence of brain chemistry alteration among substance abusers
        - ▶ A deficiency in dopamine and norepinephrine is apparent in cocaine abusers
        - ▶ A deficiency in enkephalins and endorphins has been noted in narcotics abusers and alcohol abusers
- ■ Psychological theory
    - ◆ Many substance abusers are attempting to lift underlying depression or to reduce tension, frustration, and psychic pain
    - ◆ Individuals with low self-esteem briefly feel empowered after using the substance
    - ◆ For some abusers, the substance relieves loneliness resulting from lack of meaningful relationships

---

Diagnostic criteria for substance dependence

Here are the *DSM-IV-TR* diagnostic criteria for substance dependence.

A. The person demonstrates a maladaptive pattern of substance abuse, leading to clinically significant impairment or distress.

B. The condition is manifested by three or more of the following, occurring at any time in the same 12 months:

  1. The person demonstrates evidence of tolerance, as defined by either of the following:
     a. A need for markedly increased amounts of the substance to achieve intoxication or desired effect
     b. Markedly diminished effect with continued use of the same amount of the substance
  2. The person demonstrates evidence of withdrawal, as manifested by either of the following:
     a. The characteristic withdrawal syndrome for the substance (refer to criteria A and B of the criteria sets for withdrawal from the specific substances)
     b. The need to take the same (or a closely related) substance to relieve or avoid withdrawal symptoms
  3. The substance is often taken in larger amounts or over a longer period than was intended.
  4. There is a persistent desire or unsuccessful efforts to cut down or control substance use.
  5. A great deal of time is spent in activities necessary to obtain the substance (visiting multiple doctors or driving long distances), use the substance (such as chain-smoking), or recover from its effects.
  6. Important social, occupational, or recreational activities are given up or reduced because of the substance use.
  7. The substance use is continued despite knowledge of having a persistent or recurrent physical or psychological problem that is likely to have been caused or exacerbated by the substance (for example, current cocaine use despite recognition of cocaine-induced depression, or continued drinking despite recognition that an ulcer was made worse by alcohol consumption).

Specify **with physiologic dependence** if the patient demonstrates evidence of tolerance or withdrawal (item 1 or 2 is present). *Specify* **without physiologic dependence** if the patient does not demonstrate evidence of tolerance or withdrawal (neither item 1 nor 2 is present).

Adapted from *Diagnostic and Statistical Manual of Mental Disorders,* 4th ed., text revision. Washington, D.C.: American Psychiatric Association, 2000 with permission of the publisher.

- Sociocultural theory
  - Many individuals become addicted during adolescence, when peer pressure is particularly strong
  - Substance abuse is directly linked to low socioeconomic status and racial oppression, as evidenced by high rates of abuse among Native Americans and poor Black males
  - Cultural beliefs about the responsible use of alcohol mitigate against abuse, as evidenced by the low rate of abuse among Jewish people
  - Social expectations and encouragement of consumption promote irresponsible use, as evidenced by the high rate of abuse among sociocultural groups that tolerate alcohol or drug consumption
- Behavioral-cognitive theory
  - The addicted person associates certain cues (such as the end of a workday or a weekend party) with ingestion of the substance; craving results when the person is in situations reminiscent of heavy consumption
  - Consumption provides the person with short-term rewards, reinforcing the consumption pattern

◆ The person ultimately comes to see no escape from an intolerable situation other than by ingesting one or more substances

❖ **Alcohol abuse**
- Conditions associated with alcohol abuse
  - ◆ Alcohol withdrawal syndrome
    - ▶ Develops within 4 to 12 hours of the last drink
    - ▶ Produces vivid auditory hallucinations that usually last from a few hours to a few days but may persist for weeks or months
  - ◆ Substance withdrawal delirium (alcohol)
    - ▶ Develops within 48 to 72 hours of the last drink
    - ▶ Occurs primarily in those who have been heavy drinkers for at least 5 years
    - ▶ Produces visual hallucinations, paranoia, and disorientation (see *Nursing management of substance abuse and withdrawal,* pages 98 and 99)
  - ◆ Wernicke-Korsakoff syndrome
    - ▶ Results from a deficiency in vitamin B complex (most commonly a thiamine deficiency)
    - ▶ Severely impairs cognitive functioning
    - ▶ Produces peripheral neuropathy, cerebellar ataxia, confabulation, and myopathies
    - ▶ Death can occur if thiamine replacement therapy isn't initiated immediately
- Physiologic effects of alcohol abuse
  - ◆ Cardiovascular
    - ▶ Cardiomyopathy
    - ▶ Hypertension (increased systolic pressure)
  - ◆ Gastrointestinal
    - ▶ Cancer of oral mucosa
    - ▶ Cirrhosis of the liver
    - ▶ Colitis
    - ▶ Decreased ability to absorb vitamins B_1 and B_{12}, resulting in malnutrition
    - ▶ Esophageal varices
    - ▶ Gastritis
    - ▶ Pancreatitis, acute or chronic
    - ▶ Ulcers
    - ▶ Alcoholic hepatitis
    - ▶ Portal hypertension
    - ▶ Ascites
    - ▶ Hepatic encephalopathy
  - ◆ Genitourinary
    - ▶ Impotence
    - ▶ Loss of potassium from increased urine output
    - ▶ Menstrual cycle disturbances

(Text continues on page 100.)

Nursing management of substance abuse and withdrawal

When caring for a patient who's suffering the effects of substance abuse, the nurse should be alert for signs of intoxication or withdrawal. As shown here, these signs can vary, depending on the substance ingested and the time of ingestion.

Substance	Signs of intoxication	Signs of withdrawal	Nursing implications
Alcohol (beer, wine, liquor)	Labile affect, ataxia, impaired cognition, euphoria, diplopia, dysmetria, depressed mood, flushing, dry mouth, nystagmus, slurred speech, drowsiness, sense of floating, anorexia, violence	*Stage I:* Mild tremors, diaphoresis, nausea, nervousness, increased pulse rate and blood pressure	• Monitor the patient's vital signs and behavior. • Seek a physician's order for a benzodiazepine to decrease withdrawal symptoms. • Remain with the patient. • Promote sleep and rest.
		Stage II: Moderate to severe tremors, hyperactivity, insomnia, loss of appetite, disorientation, delusions, visual hallucinations	• Administer a benzodiazepine as ordered. • Keep the environment quiet. • Remain with the patient. • Monitor vital signs. • Orient the patient to reality.
		Stage III: Persistent hallucinations, generalized tonic-clonic seizures (12 to 48 hours after last drink)	• Monitor vital signs. • Remain with the patient. • Administer anticonvulsant medication as ordered. • Offer fluids and light foods during periods of lucidity. • Keep the environment quiet and nonstimulating. • Institute seizure precautions.
		Stage IV: Alcohol withdrawal delirium, insomnia, hallucinations, tachycardia (within 3 to 5 hours after last drink)	• Remain with the patient. • Monitor vital signs. • Keep the environment quiet. • Offer food and fluids during periods of lucidity.
Opioids (morphine, heroin)	Anxiety, impaired cognition, delirium, euphoria, flushing, sense of floating, hypotonia, pinhole pupils, skin picking, sleepiness, anorexia	Tearing (lacrimation), runny nose (rhinorrhea), excessive sweating, yawning, tachycardia, fever, insomnia, muscle aches, craving, nausea or vomiting, dilated pupils, chills	• Monitor vital signs. • Remain with the patient. • Offer fluids and light foods as tolerated. • Keep the environment nondistracting and soothing. • Administer small doses of methadone, if ordered, to wean the patient.

Nursing management of substance abuse and withdrawal *(continued)*

Substance	Signs of intoxication	Signs of withdrawal	Nursing implications
Central nervous system stimulants (amphetamines, cocaine, crack)	Labile affect, anxiety, anorexia, arrhythmia, restlessness, tremors, coryza, delirium, dizziness, euphoria, skin picking, violence, hallucinations, irritability, generalized tonic-clonic seizures, dry mouth, sleep disturbance, paresthesia, dilated pupils, hyperactive reflexes, tachycardia	Depression, fatigue, agitation, suicidal thoughts, paranoia, insomnia or hypersomnia, and (with amphetamines) disorientation	• Promote sleep and rest. • Monitor vital signs. • Monitor for suicidal ideation. • Administer an antidepressant, if ordered. • Remain with a frightened or disoriented patient. • Orient the patient to reality.
Hallucinogens (lysergic acid diethylamide [LSD], phencyclidine [PCP])	*LSD or PCP:* Hyperactive reflexes, restlessness, suspiciousness, tachycardia, hallucinations, labile affect, anorexia, body image changes, hypertension, dizziness, euphoria, sense of floating *LSD only:* Anxiety, sleep disturbance, tremors, dilated pupils *PCP only:* Slurred speech, blank stare, irritability, generalized tonic-clonic seizures, nystagmus, violence, vomiting, ataxia, delirium, depressed mood, dysmetria	*LSD:* None *PCP:* Depression, lethargy, craving	• Institute safety precautions.
Cannabis (marijuana)	Slowed speech, apathy, slowed reflexes, reduced inhibitions, altered state of awareness, red eyes, dry mouth, memory loss, lethargy	Anxiety, restlessness	• Help a patient with memory loss to fill in gaps of information. • Attend to self-care needs that a lethargic or apathetic patient may have neglected.
Barbiturates and antianxiety agents (diazepam, pentobarbital)	Drowsiness, euphoria, fatigue, sense of floating, hypotonia, orthostatic hypotension, irritability, anorexia, anxiety, slurred speech, ataxia, poor memory and comprehension, seizures, delirium, depressed mood, diplopia, dizziness, dysmetria, nystagmus, violence	Nausea or vomiting, generalized malaise, tachycardia, excessive sweating, anxiety, irritability, orthostatic hypotension, insomnia, generalized tonic-clonic seizures, coarse tremors of hands, tongue, and eyelids	• Monitor vital signs. • Remain with the patient. • Promote sleep and rest. • Offer fluids and light foods as tolerated. • Administer medications, if ordered, to wean the patient. • Institute seizure precautions.

◆ Hematologic
  ▶ Anemia
  ▶ Hematomas
  ▶ Leukopenia
  ▶ Thrombocytopenia
◆ Musculoskeletal
  ▶ Fractures
  ▶ Myopathies
◆ Neurologic
  ▶ Cerebral atrophy
  ▶ Impaired cognition and memory; blackouts
  ▶ Peripheral neuropathies
  ▶ Wernicke-Korsakoff syndrome
◆ Respiratory
  ▶ Chronic obstructive pulmonary disease
  ▶ Susceptibility to chronic infections
■ Screening tests to identify alcohol abuse
  ◆ CAGE questionnaire
    ▶ Consists of four questions
      • Have you ever felt you should cut down on your drinking?
      • Have people annoyed you by criticizing your drinking?
      • Have you ever felt bad or guilty about your drinking?
      • Have you ever had a drink first thing in the morning to steady nerves or get rid of a hangover (eye-opener)?
    ▶ Indicates addiction with at least two affirmative responses
  ◆ Michigan Alcoholism Screening Test
    ▶ Consists of 26 items; points are allotted for affirmative responses
    ▶ Presumes alcoholism with four or more points (see *Michigan Alcoholism Screening Test*)
■ Continuum of alcohol consumption
  ◆ Experimental use: the first few times alcohol is ingested, the user is trying it out
  ◆ Responsible use: consumption is occasional and does no harm to the user
  ◆ Occasional misuse: consumption puts the user over the legal limit for intoxication on some occasions
  ◆ Early addiction (regular misuse): the person drinks to cope; intake is rapid; the person becomes preoccupied with alcohol, sneaks drinks, and experiences hangovers, blackouts, and personality changes
  ◆ Middle addiction (middle dependency): the person sets out to drink; begins to lie about, feel guilty about, and make excuses for drinking; has blackouts more frequently; loses friends and interests; loses control over drinking
  ◆ Late addiction (late dependency): the person can't do without alcohol; drinks until alcohol is gone, then searches for more; drinks to feel normal; alcohol becomes more important than anything in life; thinking becomes impaired; the person begins morning consumption

Michigan Alcoholism Screening Test

Many health professionals rely on the Michigan Alcoholism Screening Test to determine the nature and severity of a patient's alcohol abuse. To use this assessment tool, ask the patient the questions in the left column. For each affirmative response (except where indicated by an asterisk), assign the number of points indicated in the right column; then total the points. Generally, a score of five or more points indicates alcoholism; a four-point total suggests alcoholism; and a score of three or less indicates that the patient is not an alcoholic.

Questions	Points
1. Do you enjoy a drink now and then?	0
2. Do you feel you are a normal drinker (that is, do you drink less than or as much as most other people)?*	2
3. Have you ever awakened the morning after drinking the night before and found that you could not remember a part of the evening?	2
4. Does your spouse (or do your parents) ever worry or complain about your drinking?	1
5. Can you stop drinking without a struggle after one or two drinks?*	2
6. Do you ever feel guilty about your drinking?	1
7. Do friends and relatives think you are a normal drinker?*	2
8. Are you able to stop drinking when you want to?*	2
9. Have you ever attended a meeting of Alcoholics Anonymous (AA)?	5
10. Have you ever gotten into fights when drinking?	1
11. Has drinking ever created problems between you and your spouse (or parents)?	2
12. Has your spouse (or another family member) ever gone to anyone for help about your drinking?	2
13. Have you ever lost friends because of drinking?	2
14. Have you ever gotten into trouble at work or school because of drinking?	2
15. Have you ever lost a job because of drinking?	2
16. Have you ever neglected your obligations, your family, or your work for 2 or more days because you were drinking?	2
17. Do you drink before noon fairly often?	1
18. Have you ever been told that you have liver trouble? Cirrhosis?	2
19. After heavy drinking, have you ever had delirium tremens (DTs) or severe shaking, heard voices, or seen things that were not really there?	5
20. Have you ever gone to anyone for help about your drinking?	5
21. Have you ever been in a hospital because of drinking?	5
22. Have you ever been a patient in a psychiatric hospital or on a psychiatric ward of a general hospital when drinking was part of the problem that resulted in hospitalization?	2
23. Have you ever been seen at a psychiatric or mental health clinic or gone to any doctor, social worker, or counselor for help with an emotional problem that involved drinking?	2
24. Have you ever been arrested for driving while intoxicated?	2 each
25. Have you ever been arrested, even for a few hours, because of drunken behavior?	2 each

Adapted from Selzer, M.L. "The Michigan Alcoholism Screening Test: The Quest for a New Diagnostic Instrument," *American Journal of Psychiatry* 127(12):1653-58, 1971 with permission of the publisher.

❖ Drug abuse
- ■ Opioid (narcotic) abuse
  - ◆ Morphine, meperidine, heroin, and codeine are the most commonly abused opioids
  - ◆ Narcotic abusers quickly develop a tolerance for the narcotic, which increases the amount required to obtain the desired effect

◆ Physiologically, the person experiences a reduced ability to feel pain, along with respiratory depression, drowsiness, and a diminution in GI function

◆ Psychologically, the person experiences a sense of extreme euphoria (or "high"), apathy, impaired judgment, and detachment from reality

◆ A narcotics overdose causes respiratory and cardiovascular depression that can lead to coma and death

■ Cocaine abuse

◆ Effects are short-acting, lasting about 5 minutes when smoked as crack, 30 minutes when injected, and up to 90 minutes when inhaled

◆ Physiologically, the person experiences tachycardia, fever, and increased blood pressure and cardiac output

◆ Physiologic responses to cocaine can be severe; sudden death has been associated with cocaine use

◆ Psychologically, the drug produces a sense of high energy, extreme euphoria, and marked increase in self-confidence; these effects make the drug extremely addictive

■ Benzodiazepine abuse

◆ Initially believed to be safe, these drugs were overprescribed for many years, causing many people to become dependent

◆ Psychologically, the drugs produce euphoria, relaxation, and a sense of well-being

◆ Physiologically, the drugs produce drowsiness, unsteady gait, and impaired verbal communication

◆ Withdrawal is potentially hazardous, sometimes resulting in seizures

■ Barbiturate abuse

◆ Long used as sedatives, barbiturates cause a reaction similar to that caused by alcohol

◆ Psychologically, the drugs create euphoria, depression and, in some cases, hostile behavior

◆ Physiologically, the drugs exert a depressing effect on all body systems, especially reducing coordination

◆ Barbiturates combined with alcohol have a synergistic effect, potentially resulting in profound physiologic collapse

❖ **Effects of addiction on life**

■ Erosion of spiritual values and moral standards

■ Physical impairment, ranging from hangover to severe physiologic malfunctioning from organ damage

■ Mental deterioration, ranging from impaired judgment to severe dementia

■ Emotional symptoms, ranging from embarrassment to guilt, regret, and frequent use of defense mechanisms to justify abuse

■ Mounting family tensions as the abuser's behavior becomes more unpredictable and the family accommodates the abuser's behaviors

■ Dwindling circle of social friendships, eventually to include only fellow abusers

■ Sexual promiscuity

■ Reduction in leisure activities, with increasing amounts of time spent seeking out and consuming the substance

■ Financial problems, with increasing amounts of money diverted to procuring the substance

■ Legal difficulties as behavior deteriorates (such as driving under the influence or stealing to maintain the habit)

■ Occupational problems, with poor quality of work and unreliability sometimes resulting in termination

❖ **Resources for abusers and their families**
   ■ Support for abusers
      ◆ Alcoholics Anonymous
         ▮ Self-help group based on a 12-step program designed to help the person remain abstinent
         ▮ Groups may be open (anyone may attend) or closed (only alcoholics may attend)
      ◆ Cocaine Anonymous
      ◆ Narcotics Anonymous
      ◆ Pills Anonymous
      ◆ Women for Sobriety: a group for female alcoholics
      ◆ Rational Recovery: a group for alcoholism
   ■ Support for families
      ◆ Adult Children of Alcoholics (ACoA): a group for adults who need to work through unresolved issues related to growing up in an alcoholic home
      ◆ Al-Anon: a support group for family members and friends of alcoholics; the group teaches its members about the disease of alcoholism and how to let the addicted member become responsible for self
      ◆ Alateen: a support group for children ages 10 to 17; in this group, children of alcoholics can share experiences and learn how to deal with their alcoholic parents
      ◆ Children Are People: a group for school-age children with an alcoholic family member
      ◆ Families Anonymous: a support group for parents of children who abuse substances
      ◆ Nar-Anon: a group for families of narcotic addicts

❖ **Interventions in addiction disorders**
   ■ Therapeutic intervention
      ◆ This is a technique for confronting abusers with their maladaptive behavior
      ◆ The goal is to get the abuser into a treatment program
      ◆ A therapeutic intervention consists of two important meetings

▶ In the first session, people who are important to the abuser (spouse, children, boss, friends, physician) meet with an intervention counselor to plan the intervention; during this meeting, which the abuser doesn't attend, the group agrees on what to say and how to say it

▶ During the second session, with the abuser present, those assembled express their concern for the abuser; share examples of the abuser's behavior, thus acting as a mirror to the abuser; and explain the consequences of not seeking immediate treatment (for instance, "You can't come home" or "You won't have a job")

◆ A carefully planned therapeutic intervention negates the abuser's main weapons — denial and manipulation — because all significant others are assembled in the same room

■ Detoxification
   ◆ Physical withdrawal from a chemical substance requires medical supervision to prevent physiologic collapse
   ◆ The purpose of detoxification is to prevent physical and emotional complications while the body undergoes withdrawal from the substance

■ In-facility treatment
   ◆ The abuser resides at a special facility for a specified time, commonly from 21 to 30 days
   ◆ Education about substance abuse and group and individual therapy are emphasized
   ◆ In-facility treatment typically follows detoxification

■ Day treatment
   ◆ The abuser stays at a treatment center during the day for individual and group activities
   ◆ Areas of emphasis include abstinence and change of lifestyle to maintain recovery
   ◆ Day treatment provides a support system during early recovery

■ Halfway house
   ◆ A halfway house provides a support system for addicts during the first few months of recovery (early recovery)
   ◆ The emphasis is on assuming responsibility for one's well-being
   ◆ Maintenance of the house is the responsibility of the residents
   ◆ Most residents are expected to find employment and adjust to living drug-free in the community

■ Alcoholics Anonymous
   ◆ AA emphasizes accepting and practicing the 12 steps for successful recovery from alcohol addiction
   ◆ New recoverers are encouraged to seek a sponsor to whom they can turn for support at any time
   ◆ Meetings are held daily, and members are advised to attend as many meetings weekly as needed to maintain sobriety
   ◆ Membership and attendance at meetings are strictly voluntary

◆ Because recovery is considered a lifelong process, many members attend meetings throughout their lives
■ Group therapy
◆ Group therapy enables the recovering addict to get feedback from peers
◆ It provides the addict with a temporary support system
■ Family therapy
◆ Because the addiction of one member disrupts the entire family and can lead to dysfunction, the primary emphasis is on helping the family unit to remain intact if family members desire it
◆ Members learn how to take care of themselves by setting realistic boundaries for behavior and by respecting the personal belongings of other members
◆ A specially trained family therapist assists members by discussing such issues as codependency and by encouraging reenactments of family roles
■ Marital therapy
◆ In marital therapy, the spouses identify the ways in which addiction has affected their marriage
◆ They explore options for remaining together or separating
◆ The therapist aids the couple in their attempts to develop viable solutions to their problems
■ Behavior therapy
◆ In aversion therapy, the abuser experiences a negative sanction, such as vomiting, if consumption of alcohol begins
  ◗ Disulfiram (Antabuse) is commonly prescribed for alcoholics during early recovery
  ◗ Because alcohol interacts with the drug to produce violent vomiting, the person shouldn't drink alcohol or use alcohol-containing products (such as aftershave, liquid cough and cold medicines, rubbing alcohol, mouthwash, nail polish remover, and cologne) while taking disulfiram
◆ When stressed or tense, the person can use relaxation techniques, which dissipate the automatic urge to consume the substance
◆ Relapse prevention involves teaching the person to recognize and avoid the cues that lead to consumption; in some instances, old friends must be avoided and new friendships cultivated
◆ Assertiveness training shows the person how to feel empowered without relying on a substance
■ Employee assistance programs
◆ Business firms have set up special programs that provide professional care to employees who suffer from substance dependence
◆ Education and support from coworkers and the employer are available to the employee during recovery; responsibility in the workplace is emphasized

❖ **Levels of addiction prevention**
   ■ *Primary prevention* focuses on preventing substance abuse, usually through education programs aimed at children and adolescents
   ■ *Secondary prevention* focuses on early identification of and intervention with substance abusers to prevent recurrence
   ■ *Tertiary prevention* focuses on rehabilitation to prevent recurrence (see *Nursing management of substance abuse and withdrawal,* pages 98 and 99)

Clinical situation

Jim Curry, age 41, is brought to the emergency department by his girl-friend, who says Jim vomited what looked like coffee grounds about 20 minutes earlier. The emergency department physician decides to admit him to the hospital for diagnostic testing. When Jim arrives on your nursing unit, you notice that he looks older than his stated age. He's pale and diaphoretic. He's 5'10" tall and weighs 150 lb (68 kg). Your assessment reveals the following: temperature, 100° F (37.8° C); pulse rate, 120 beats/minute; blood pressure, 146/100 mm Hg; clear lung sounds; slightly distended abdomen; slightly yellow sclera.

As part of your nursing assessment, you ask Jim about his use of substances. He states that he smokes two packs of cigarettes per day, drinks four to five cups of coffee in the morning only, and consumes "a little beer" every day. When you ask Jim to quantify "a little beer," he says, "Maybe a can or two." He begins to squirm when you ask whether he uses other substances. "I don't do any hard stuff. I might smoke pot once in a while—just to mellow out. Pot isn't harmful, you know. Most people just don't understand how it works."

Because Jim says he feels nauseated, you decide to let him rest. You tell him that you'll be leaving soon and that another nurse will be caring for him during the evening. At 10 p.m., Jim asks the evening nurse for "something for my nerves." Jim is mildly tremulous and perspiring. His pulse rate is 130 beats/minute, and his blood pressure is 158/120 mm Hg. Suspecting that Jim might be experiencing early-stage alcohol withdrawal, the nurse confers with the supervisor, who arranges to transfer Jim immediately to the hospital's detoxification unit.

Assessment (nursing behaviors and rationales)

1. Assess changes in Jim's physiologic status. *Increased pulse rate and blood pressure signal stage I of alcohol withdrawal syndrome.*

2. Assess Jim's level of orientation. *Fluctuating levels of orientation signal stage II withdrawal. Preventing late-stage alcohol withdrawal syndrome will be a top priority.*

3. Assess Jim for anxiety and alcohol hallucinosis. *Physical signs resulting from withdrawal can produce moderate to severe anxiety levels. Withdrawal causes the patient to misperceive external stimuli, resulting in misinterpretation of what's really happening (hallucinosis).*

4. Assess Jim's nutritional status. *Drinking bouts may have caused the patient to develop poor eating habits, causing vitamin deficiencies and electrolyte imbalances.*

Nursing diagnoses

- Risk for injury related to confusion and unsteadiness
- Imbalanced nutrition: Less than body requirements related to poor eating habits
- Disturbed sleep pattern related to alcohol withdrawal

Planning and goals

- Jim won't injure himself while on the detoxification unit.
- He won't experience stage II withdrawal.
- He'll reestablish a nutritious diet.
- He'll be less confused and will have fewer misperceptions of external stimuli.

Implementation (nursing behaviors and rationales)

1. Provide one-on-one monitoring as long as Jim's condition is unstable. *One-on-one monitoring ensures the continuous assessment necessary for calibration of medication to control withdrawal and to provide a safe environment.*
2. Administer medication (usually a benzodiazepine) as prescribed. Jim's physician has prescribed lorazepam (Ativan) 2 mg every 8 hours on the first day, 1 mg every 8 hours on the second day, and 0.5 mg every 8 hours on the third day, along with thiamine 100 mg I.M. for 3 days. *Lorazepam is administered to prevent acute alcohol withdrawal syndrome. Because this patient may have liver damage, lorazepam is the benzodiazepine of choice because of its short half-life. Thiamine promotes the body's ability to utilize carbohydrates fully.*
3. Document Jim's response to lorazepam. If the ordered dosage isn't effective, the physician will need to increase it. *Preventing second-stage withdrawal is necessary for the patient's safety.*
4. Maintain a quiet, peaceful environment by speaking softly, dimming the lights in Jim's room, and screening out noises. *A quiet, peaceful environment promotes rest and enhances the medication's sedative qualities.*
5. While acknowledging his feelings and experiences, reassure Jim that visual hallucinations (such as animals or insects) aren't real. Provide emotional support. *Emphasizing reality, acknowledging the patient's feelings, and providing empathy are crucial to helping the patient through the first phase of alcohol withdrawal syndrome.*

Evaluation

- Jim completes detoxification without incident.
- He doesn't experience second-stage withdrawal.

Clinical situation (continued)

Before Jim Curry leaves the detoxification unit, his physician, girlfriend, and two children participate in a therapeutic intervention with him. As a result of the intervention, Jim reluctantly agrees to transfer to an inpatient treatment setting.

Medical records sent from the hospital to the inpatient treatment setting reveal that Jim's hemoglobin (Hb) level was 10 g/dl. Toxicology screening showed that when Jim entered the hospital, his blood alcohol level was 0.23 and his urine was positive for cannabis. Jim's gamma-glutamyl transpeptidase test reveals liver damage.

On his 1st day in the treatment setting, Jim completes the CAGE questionnaire, answering the second and fourth questions affirmatively. However, Jim is adamant that his alcohol consumption isn't unreasonable. "After all, I only drink beer," he says.

During the next 2 weeks, Jim attends multiple individual and group sessions as well as classes in which the disease of alcoholism is explained. Jim reluctantly participates in these activities. He manages self-care but has lost 3 lb (1 kg) because he "just isn't hungry." Jim's counselor learns that Jim consumes up to 12 cans of beer daily and uses cannabis three times weekly. Jim states that he has always been able to drink more than most people. When asked about hangovers, Jim replies that he used to get them but hasn't had any bad hangovers for at least 5 years. When asked about family history, Jim reveals that his father, uncles, and grandfather were "heavy drinkers." He says his mother never consumed alcohol.

Assessment (nursing behaviors and rationales)

1. Monitor Jim's physical condition, especially noting Hb level, weight and appetite, and signs of jaundice. *Medical evidence proves that the patient's prolonged use of alcohol has damaged his body. Physical problems must be corrected to ensure the patient's physical well-being and to prevent further damage. Lower-level needs must be met first.*

2. Assess Jim's use of denial. *The nurse must determine the patient's progress toward understanding that he has an alcohol problem and that he must take responsibility for his recovery.*

Nursing diagnoses

- Ineffective denial related to the patient's consumption pattern
- Imbalanced nutrition: Less than body requirements related to lack of appetite, gastric ulcer, and deteriorating physical health

Planning and goals

- Jim will state at least three effects that alcohol has had on his body.
- He'll consume nutritional foods offered and will attain a weight of at least 150 lb (68 kg).

Implementation (nursing behaviors and rationales)

1. Explain the alcohol-use continuum, and ask Jim to place himself along that continuum (see "Continuum of alcohol consumption," page 100). *This activity will encourage the patient to look objectively at how alcohol has affected his life.*

2. Review the CAGE questionnaire with Jim. *Discussing how others view the patient's alcohol consumption and how he needs alcohol early in the day chips away at the wall of denial he has erected.*

3. Have Jim attend meetings with alcohol-abuse peers who have moved beyond denial. *What peers say commonly carries more weight than what health care professionals say.*

4. Provide Jim with a menu of nutritious foods, and ask him to indicate his preferences. *An appropriate diet will help correct nutritional deficiencies. The patient will be more likely to follow the diet if it contains foods that he enjoys.*

5. Offer small quantities of nutritious food every 3 hours. *A patient who doesn't feel well usually can't a lot at one time. Keeping food in the stomach will absorb gastric acids. The patient's ability to maintain a healthy weight depends on the amount of food he ingests.*

Evaluation

- Jim recognizes the effects that alcohol has had on his body.
- He weighs 151 lb (68 kg) and consumes the food offered to him.

Clinical situation (continued)

Jim Curry has been in treatment for 16 days. Today, during a rather intense group session, Jim tells the group about his two failed marriages, his strained relationships with his 14- and 17-year-old children, and numerous jobs lost over the past 20 years. He further relates how he contracted genital herpes 5 years ago during a blackout. With great feeling, Jim says he regrets the years he has wasted, the hardships he has imposed on others, and his flagrant disregard of the values he once held dear. He shakes his head sadly and says, "I don't know if I can ever be forgiven for all the damage I've done."

Assessment (nursing behaviors and rationales)

1. Assess Jim's coping skills. *The patient has used alcohol and marijuana in the past to cope with stress. If he has no legitimate coping skills, he'll need to learn new ones to prevent relapse or suicide.*

2. Assess Jim's support system, including spiritual values. *Without an adequate support system, the potential for relapse increases.*

3. Assess what Jim wants to accomplish sober that he couldn't accomplish while abusing alcohol and marijuana. *This provides the patient with structure during recovery and allows the nurse to evaluate how well the patient can set attainable goals.*

4. Assess Jim's sexual practices and his knowledge about sexually transmitted diseases (STDs). *A patient with genital herpes must have accurate information to control the contagious disease. The patient also is at risk for contracting other STDs.*

Nursing diagnoses

- Dysfunctional family processes: Alcoholism related to impaired judgment and developmental immaturity
- Dysfunctional grieving related to engaging in behaviors contrary to the patient's core value system
- Ineffective sexuality patterns related to contracting an STD

Planning and goals

- Jim will identify behaviors appropriate for parenting, intimate sexual relationships, employment, and social relationships.
- He'll identify the core values most important to him.
- He'll describe how to protect others from contracting genital herpes and how to protect himself against other STDs.

Implementation (nursing behaviors and rationales)

1. Enroll Jim in parenting classes. *These classes will enable the patient to develop effective parenting skills, thereby enhancing his ability to relate with his children in a mutually rewarding way.*

2. Have Jim attend an ACoA meeting. *In this group, the patient will learn how his father's alcoholism affected him as a child and as an adult. Additionally, he'll have opportunities to build a support system and to relate to others with similar experiences.*

3. Role-play various life situations with Jim, focusing on situations that would create stress in everyday life. *The patient's past coping skills have proved to be limited and ineffective; role-playing is a safe way for the patient to develop the new skills he'll need to remain sober.*

4. Have Jim attend AA at least three times a week during the first few months of recovery. *Adequate support can help prevent relapse, which is more likely to occur during the first year of recovery than at any other time. AA is a spiritually based self-help group that will assist the patient in reestablishing spiritual balance in his life and provide him with emotional support. He'll learn how to make peace with himself and those important to him.*

5. Teach Jim the importance of practicing safer sex, including condom use and avoidance of anal sex and body fluid intake. Explain that abstinence from sex is the only certain way to prevent the spread of STDs and that maintaining a monogamous relationship is safer than engaging in sex with multiple partners. *Knowledge of safer sexual practices contributes to the well-being of the patient and his sexual partners.*

6. Teach Jim how to manage genital herpes if he doesn't already know how. *This is important to the patient's physical and social well-being.*

7. Have Jim role-play how to tell his sex partners that he has genital herpes. *The patient will be more likely to inform future partners if he has practiced how to do this and is comfortable with it.*

Evaluation

- Jim enrolls in a class for parents of teenagers.
- He has found a job in his area of expertise.
- He has developed friendships with others in his ACoA and AA groups and plans to join them on social occasions.
- He's learning how to accept and practice the 12 steps of the recovery program. He says he feels good about the progress he's beginning to make.
- He has attended classes on human sexuality and can describe safer sexual practices. He has discussed his herpes with his girlfriend. They practice safer sex, and she remains free of the disease.
- He and his girlfriend have elected to attend two to four sessions with a counselor to sort out their relationship.

Review questions

1. After several days of heavy drinking, a patient is brought into the emergency department at midnight and is taken to an intensive care step-down unit. When should the nurses expect the patient to show signs and symptoms of alcohol withdrawal syndrome?

○ **A.** Around 4 a.m. to noon

○ **B.** Around 4 p.m. to midnight

○ **C.** Between 24 and 48 hours after admission

○ **D.** Between 48 and 72 hours after admission

Correct answer: A Acute alcohol withdrawal syndrome begins within 4 to 12 hours of the last drink and may last for several days, weeks, or months. Options B, C, and D are too late for the symptoms to begin occurring.

2. A patient is admitted to the hospital with a drug overdose, and family members are uncertain what the patient was taking. The nurse notes the following symptoms: tachycardia, fever, increased blood pressure, and increased cardiac output. Based on these symptoms, what drug would the nurse suspect the patient was using?

○ **A.** Heroin

○ **B.** Cocaine

○ **C.** Benzodiazepines

○ **D.** Barbiturates

Correct answer: B The assessment findings of the nurse all indicate cocaine abuse. Signs of heroin abuse include reduced ability to feel pain, respiratory depression, drowsiness, and decreased GI functioning. Signs of benzodiazepine abuse include drowsiness, unsteady gait, and impaired verbal communication. Signs of barbiturate abuse include a depressing effect on all body systems, especially reducing coordination.

3. The school nurse in a public high school is approached by parents who believe their child is abusing drugs and alcohol. The parents list the signs and symptoms to support this suspicion. The school nurse notes no problems at school; however, the student has skipped school on occasion. The parents have talked to their child without success and are asking for some help. Which group should the nurse recommend to the parents?

○ **A.** Alcoholics Anonymous

○ **B.** Children Are People

○ **C.** Alateen

○ **D.** Families Anonymous

Correct answer: D Families Anonymous is for parents of children who abuse substances. Because the parents have had no success in talking with the child, they need a support group for themselves. The parents can seek a group for the child when he's ready for help. Alcoholics Anonymous is for the alcoholic who's ready for help. Alateen and Children Are People are support groups for children of adults who are substance abusers.

4. A patient who feels drowsy, euphoric, and fatigued is admitted to the substance abuse unit after gradually increasing his dosage of diazepam (Valium). The nursing implications for this patient include placing the patient on which precaution?

○ **A.** Seizure

○ **B.** Suicide

○ **C.** Homicide

○ **D.** Elopement

Correct answer: A Patients who have overdosed on barbiturates or antianxiety agents are at risk for seizure activity as the medication clears from their body. The other precautions — suicide, homicide, and elopement — aren't appropriate unless the patient has mentioned them.

CHAPTER 11

Adjustment disorders

❖ Overview

- An adjustment disorder is characterized by a maladaptive reaction to a psychosocial stressor that can be readily identified
  - ◆ The reaction is considered maladaptive under certain circumstances
    - ❭ Social or occupational (including school) functioning is markedly impaired
    - ❭ The symptoms exhibited are exaggerated beyond the usual expected response to the severity of the stressor
    - ❭ The response doesn't meet the criteria for any other mental disorder and is neither an isolated incident nor uncomplicated bereavement (see *Diagnostic criteria for adjustment disorders,* page 114)
  - ◆ The maladaptive reaction occurs within 3 months after the onset of the stressor and can't have lasted longer than 6 months
  - ◆ An adjustment disorder may be characterized as chronic if the disturbance lasts longer than 6 months. Typically, such symptoms are in response to a chronic stressor such as a debilitating physical illness
- Clinicians recognize six types of adjustment disorder, classified by the predominant symptom or group of symptoms displayed (see *Types of adjustment disorders,* page 115)
  - ◆ Although many of the types described are similar to other psychiatric diagnoses, they're only partial syndromes of other mental disorders
  - ◆ For example, adjustment disorder with depressed mood and adjustment disorder with anxious mood aren't severe enough to be diagnosed as depression or anxiety
- Behavioral reactions to stress are expected to remit soon after the stressor ceases or, in cases of continued stress, when a new level of adaptation is reached
- Genetic factors may dispose an individual to maladaptive response to stress
- Chronic disorders, such as mental retardation, may increase the likelihood of a maladaptive stress response

❖ Theoretical perspectives

- Biological theory
  - ◆ Problems result from biochemical imbalances in the brain

---

Diagnostic criteria for adjustment disorders

Here are the *DSM-IV-TR* diagnostic criteria for adjustment disorders.

A. The development of emotional or behavioral symptoms in response to an identifiable stressor occurring within 3 months of the onset of the stressor

B. These symptoms or behaviors are clinically significant as evidenced by either of the following:
1. Marked distress that is in excess of what would be expected from exposure to the stressor
2. Significant impairment in social or occupational (academic) functioning

C. The stress-related disturbance does not meet the criteria for another specific Axis I disorder and is not merely an exacerbation of a preexisting Axis I or Axis II disorder.

D. The symptoms do not represent bereavement.

E. After the stressor (or its consequences) has terminated, the symptoms do not persist for more than an additional 6 months.

Specify **acute** if the disturbance lasts less than 6 months; **chronic** if it lasts for 6 months or longer.

Adapted from *Diagnostic and Statistical Manual of Mental Disorders,* 4th ed., text revision. Washington, D.C.: American Psychiatric Association, 2000 with permission of the publisher.

◆ The midbrain releases norepinephrine, which causes severe anxiety (see chapter 3, Human development)

■ Psychodynamic theory
  ◆ Hidden psychological conflicts cause anxiety
  ◆ This stimulates a maladaptive response to stress in a person who:
    ▶ Can't complete appropriate developmental tasks
    ▶ Has unmet dependency needs
    ▶ Is fixated in an earlier developmental level
    ▶ Has retarded ego development

■ Interpersonal theory
  ◆ Problems result when a person's expectations or needs aren't met in interpersonal relationships with significant others
  ◆ Unsatisfactory early interpersonal relationships (for instance, early separation from one's mother) can lead to problems with adjustment later in life

■ Behavioral theory
  ◆ Maladaptive behavior is learned
  ◆ Negative learning patterns experienced by the person have impeded the development of self-esteem and effective coping skills

❖ **General nursing assessments**
  ■ Assess the time, duration, and nature of the stressor
    ◆ The patient usually reports a psychosocial stressor occurring in the 3 months before the onset of symptoms
    ◆ If symptoms last longer than 6 months, another mental disorder should be considered

Types of adjustment disorders

Here are the six types of adjustment disorders as classified by *DSM-IV-TR*.

Adjustment Disorder with Anxiety

Predominant manifestations include such symptoms as nervousness, worry, and jitteriness.

Adjustment Disorder with Depressed Mood

Predominant manifestations include such symptoms as depressed mood, tearfulness, and feelings of hopelessness.

Adjustment Disorder with Disturbance of Conduct

Predominant manifestation is conduct that violates either the rights of others or major age-appropriate societal norms and rules (for example, truancy, vandalism, reckless driving, fighting, or defaulting on legal responsibilities). The major differential is with conduct disorder or antisocial personality disorder.

Adjustment Disorder with Mixed Disturbance of Emotions and Conduct

Predominant manifestations include emotional symptoms (such as depression or anxiety) and disturbance of conduct (see above).

Adjustment Disorder with Mixed Anxiety and Depressed Mood

Predominant manifestation is a combination of depression and anxiety or other emotions (such as an adolescent who, after moving away from home and parental supervision, reacts with ambivalence, depression, anger, and signs of increased dependence). The major differential is with depressive and anxiety disorders.

Adjustment Disorder Unspecified

Disorders involving maladaptive reactions to psychosocial stressors that are not classifiable as specific types of adjustment disorder.

Adapted from *Diagnostic and Statistical Manual of Mental Disorders,* 4th ed., text revision, Washington, D.C.: American Psychiatric Association, 2000 with permission of the publisher.

◆ The symptoms may stem from a single stressor (such as loss of a job) or from multiple stressors (such as business difficulties or marital problems)

◆ Some stressors are easily identified (divorce or the death of a loved one), but others are less evident (going away to school, leaving the parental home, or other developmental milestones)

◆ The stressor may be recurrent (such as a seasonal business crisis) or continuous (such as poverty, chronic illness, a natural disaster, strained family relationships, or religious or racial prejudice)

■ Assess any impairment in social or occupational functioning for symptoms beyond the normal and expected reactions to the stressor

◆ The patient appears tearful and jittery

◆ The patient expresses anger inappropriately through fighting, vandalism, or reckless driving
◆ School or work performance declines
◆ Use or abuse of psychoactive substances increases
◆ Complaints of headache, backache, and fatigue arise

■ Assess for feelings of inadequacy, low self-esteem, and difficulty adapting to change

■ Assess the patient's pre-illness ability to cope with day-to-day problems

❖ Selected nursing diagnoses

■ Anxiety related to loss of control over life
■ Impaired adjustment related to recent change in life
■ Ineffective coping related to low self-esteem
■ Situational low self-esteem related to feelings of inadequacy
■ Ineffective role performance related to inability to solve problems
■ Powerlessness related to inability to cope
■ Dysfunctional grieving related to real or perceived loss
■ Risk for self-directed violence related to overwhelming feelings of worthlessness
■ Risk for other-directed violence related to maladaptive coping

❖ Psychotherapeutic goals and treatments

■ Most people with an adjustment disorder are treated on an outpatient basis; treatment depends on the symptoms exhibited

■ Priorities include providing for safety needs, lessening anxiety, and identifying problem-solving and coping mechanisms

■ Treatment shouldn't last longer than is necessary to relieve symptoms

■ Treatment goals include restoring the patient's level of functioning to a pre-illness level and promoting behavioral changes to strengthen that part of the patient's personality still vulnerable to stress

■ Individual psychotherapy is the most common treatment for adjustment disorders

◆ Its goal is to replace the patient's maladaptive response with a more effective one

◆ Three widely used types of psychotherapy are psychodynamic therapy, behavioral therapy, and family therapy

▶ Psychodynamic therapy
• The patient's problem results from negative self-image, early psychological trauma, or inadequate personality development
• The therapist uses supportive and expressive psychodynamic techniques to help the patient resolve the problem

▶ Behavioral therapy
• The patient's problem results from patterns of maladaptive responses to situations

- Coaching, modeling, and reinforcement schedules are some of the psychotherapeutic techniques used to help the patient correct ineffective responses to stress

  ▶ Family therapy
    - This type of therapy directs treatment away from the patient and toward the patient's family unit
    - Its goal is to change the social network function

❖ **General nursing interventions**

  ■ Monitor for danger toward self or others
    ◆ Ask the patient direct questions about any intent, plan, and means to hurt others or self
    ◆ Provide a safe environment, placing potentially harmful objects out of reach

  ■ Help the patient identify thoughts and feelings associated with the change in life or current situational crisis
    ◆ Encourage the patient to express feelings, including sadness and anger
    ◆ Explore how to handle frustration or pent-up anger in socially acceptable ways (walking briskly, engaging in a sporting event, hitting a punching bag)

  ■ Teach the patient relaxation techniques, and have the patient practice them under your supervision

  ■ Determine which stage of grief (and associated behaviors) the patient may be experiencing; teach the patient about these stages and behaviors (see chapter 3, Human development)

  ■ Help the patient determine aspects of personal life still under the patient's control
    ◆ Encourage the patient to perform self-care, to set goals, and to make independent decisions
    ◆ Help the patient identify methods of coping or problem solving that proved successful in the past
    ◆ Assist the patient in using the problem-solving process to explore alternatives and to select more adaptive strategies of coping with stress

  ■ Refer the patient to an appropriate support group, such as Alcoholics Anonymous or a bereavement group

Clinical situation

Pamela Jones, age 32, is a well-groomed legal secretary who comes to the outpatient clinic where you're on duty. She tells you that she has come on the advice of a coworker. She has been experiencing frequent bouts of crying and states that she feels as if she's "unlikable." She has canceled all of her usual social engagements and is no longer attending her aerobics class, which she previously enjoyed. Pamela states that her symptoms began about 1 month ago, after she discovered that Tom, a man she had been dating (and had expected to marry), was married and no longer wanted to see her.

Assessment (nursing behaviors and rationales)

1. Conduct a health history and physical examination. Question Pamela about alcohol and drug use, and pay special attention to current eating habits. *Any deterioration in physical health needs attention, and physical causes for symptoms must be ruled out. Severe depression can lead to changes in eating and sleeping patterns; patients typically use psychoactive substances as a coping mechanism in stressful situations.*

2. Conduct a psychosocial assessment to assess suicide potential, available social supports, occupational and financial stressors, and previous losses. Determine which coping skills the patient uses when under stress. Reinforce those coping skills that have been successfully used in the past. *A psychosocial assessment assists in determining the severity of the patient's reaction to the situation, along with patient strengths that may be useful in establishing a treatment plan.*

3. Determine the patient's perception of the situation. *The nurse must understand how the patient perceives the problem in order to establish a patient-specific treatment plan.*

Nursing diagnoses

- Dysfunctional grieving related to loss of a lover
- Ineffective coping related to a situational crisis
- Impaired social interaction related to negative self-image

Planning and goals

- Pamela Jones will express her thoughts and feelings about this loss to her close friends.
- She'll identify alternate coping skills to handle stress.
- She'll increase socialization and effectively use social support systems that are available to her.

Implementation (nursing behaviors and rationales)

1. Actively involve Pamela in the physical and psychosocial assessment. *This not only provides the data necessary to plan care but also lets the patient know that, as an active participant in her treatment, she has some control over the situation.*

2. Help Pamela identify her thoughts and feelings about the dissolution of her relationship with Tom, including negative and positive aspects of the change. *The patient may need help in viewing the change objectively because the change can have both positive and negative consequences. Her perception of the event is particularly important and needs to be explored in relation to the actual event.*

3. Encourage Pamela to express openly any anger or sadness. *This allows the patient to acknowledge her feelings and begin to deal with them. The nurse's* *acceptance of these expressions helps the patient recognize that anger and sadness are normal rather than "bad."*

4. Explore alternative physical outlets that Pamela can rely on to diffuse anger and hostility. *Physical exercise provides a safe and effective way to release pent-up emotions.*

5. Explain the stages of grief to Pamela, including the behaviors commonly associated with each stage. *Grieving over the loss of a close relationship is normal and socially accepted. Knowing this may help relieve some of the anxiety and guilt that these responses commonly generate.*

6. Encourage Pamela to review her relationship with Tom. With sensitivity and support, help her to examine the reality of a romantic situation in which one partner makes misrepresentations. *The patient must give up idealized perceptions and be able to accept both positive and negative aspects of the situation before she can complete the grieving process.*

7. Assist Pamela in identifying areas of strength and previous coping abilities. *Focusing on past success enhances the patient's self-esteem and provides a blueprint for resolving the current crisis.*

8. Teach Pamela to solve problems one step at a time. *Patients benefit from learning the steps of a logical and orderly process to solving problems. Recognition of personal control, however minimal, diminishes the sense of powerlessness and promotes a positive self-image.*

9. Encourage Pamela to discuss the situation with a trusted friend. *Interacting with an important person in the patient's life limits opportunities for isolation. Additionally, feedback from peers may help the patient correct misperceptions of the event and learn new coping behaviors.*

10. Explore Pamela's social support system with her. *Discussing available support will empower the patient to seek socialization.*

Evaluation

- Pamela Jones remained in therapy for 10 weeks.
- She resumed social contacts with friends and returned to her aerobics class.
- Confiding in her best friend, Pamela was able to express her anger at Tom's deception and her sadness about the loss of a possible marriage partner.

Review questions

1. An adjustment disorder is considered maladaptive when:

   ○ **A.** social or occupational functioning is markedly impaired.

   ○ **B.** symptoms exhibited are the usual expected response to the stressor.

   ○ **C.** the response also meets criteria for another mental disorder.

   ○ **D.** the reaction occurs longer than 12 months after the incident.

Correct answer: A An adjustment disorder is maladaptive when the functioning of the individual is markedly impaired and the symptoms are exaggerated beyond the severity of the stressor. The symptoms commonly occur within 3 months after onset of the stressor.

2. An adolescent who reacts with ambivalence, depression, anger, and signs of increased dependence after moving away from home may be experiencing an adjustment disorder with:

○ **A.** disturbance of conduct.

○ **B.** mixed disturbance of emotions and conduct.

○ **C.** mixed anxiety and depressed mood.

○ **D.** manifestations of anxiety.

Correct answer: C Predominant manifestations of adjustment disorder with mixed anxiety and depressed mood include a combination of depression and anxiety or other emotions.

3. Which of the following theoretical perspectives applies to an adjustment disorder resulting from problems occurring when a person's expectations or needs aren't met in relationships with significant others?

○ **A.** Behavioral theory

○ **B.** Interpersonal theory

○ **C.** Psychodynamic theory

○ **D.** Biological theory

Correct answer: B The interpersonal theory states that unsatisfactory early interpersonal relationships can lead to adjustment problems later in life. The behavioral theory states that maladaptive behavior is learned. These negative learning patterns impede a person's development of self-esteem and effective coping skills. The psychodynamic theory suggests that hidden psychological conflicts cause anxiety. Such conflicts stimulate a maladaptive response to stress. The biological theory examines the physiologic nature of the disturbance.

4. Treatment for the patient with adjustment disorder includes:

○ **A.** inpatient treatment.

○ **B.** extended follow-up.

○ **C.** individual psychotherapy.

○ **D.** antipsychotic agents.

Correct answer: C Individual psychotherapy is the most common treatment for adjustment disorders. Treatments are on an outpatient basis and usually last no longer than is necessary to relieve symptoms. Inpatient treatment and extended follow-up aren't indicated in adjustment disorders. Antipsychotic agents are usually not necessary.

5. Which of the following nursing interventions should take precedence for the patient with an adjustment disorder?

○ **A.** Providing a safe environment

○ **B.** Encouraging expression of feelings

○ **C.** Reviewing relaxation techniques

○ **D.** Helping the patient identify methods of coping

Correct answer: A   Because the patient with an adjustment disorder can be a danger to self or others, providing a safe environment is an essential nursing intervention. Monitoring should include asking the patient direct questions regarding injury to self or others, and the nurse should place potentially harmful objects out of the patient's reach. After establishing a safe environment, the nurse can then encourage the patient to express feelings, identify methods of coping, and practice relaxation techniques.

Dissociative disorders

❖ **Overview**
- Dissociation is a psychobiological activation of altered states of consciousness serving to protect individuals from overwhelming psychological trauma
- Dissociative disorders are characterized by a sudden disruption in consciousness, memory, identity, or perception
- Severe anxiety and psychic conflict are common precursors, and sometimes a dissociative disorder develops after a major trauma that has caused the victim to fear for his life
- Although dissociative disorders are uncommon, their occurrence produces dramatic disruptions of the person's personality

❖ **Dissociative identity disorder**
- Characteristics
  - ◆ Two or more distinct personalities, or personality states (generally referred to as "alters"), existing within the same person
    - ❯ At least two of the personalities take full control of the person's behavior at various times
    - ❯ Each of the personalities, or personality states, may have a distinct identity, self-image, and history
    - ❯ The transition from one personality to another is commonly triggered by psychosocial stress; the transition usually occurs within seconds to minutes
    - ❯ The personalities usually are aware of some or all of the others in varying degrees
    - ❯ The patient may report memory gaps or lost periods of time during which another personality is in control
  - ◆ Self-mutilation and suicidal and aggressive behavior
  - ◆ History of frequent admissions to a psychiatric facility
  - ◆ History of physical or sexual abuse or severe emotional trauma sometime during childhood
- Criteria for medical diagnosis (see the diagnostic criteria for dissociative identity disorder)
- Treatment (aims to reintegrate the personalities into one person who can function effectively in society)

Diagnostic criteria for dissociative identity disorders

Here are the *DSM-IV-TR* diagnostic criteria for the dissociative disorders discussed in this chapter.

Dissociative identity disorder

A. The person has two or more distinct identities or personality states (each with its own relatively enduring pattern of perceiving, relating to, and thinking about the environment and self).
B. At least two of these identities or personality states recurrently take control of the person's behavior.
C. The person cannot recall important personal information that is too extensive to be explained by ordinary forgetfulness.
D. The disturbance is not due to the direct physiologic effects of a substance (for example, blackouts or chaotic behavior during alcohol intoxication) or a general medical condition (such as complex partial seizures). *Note:* In children, the symptoms are not attributable to imaginary playmates or other fantasy play.

Dissociative fugue

A. The predominant disturbance is sudden, unexpected travel away from home or one's customary place of work, with inability to recall one's past.
B. The disturbance is marked by confusion about personal identity or assumption of a new identity (partial or complete).
C. The disturbance does not occur exclusively during the course of dissociative identity disorder and is not due to the direct physiologic effects of a substance (such as a drug of abuse or a medication) or a general medical condition (such as temporal lobe epilepsy).
D. The symptoms cause clinically significant distress or impairment in social, occupational, or other important areas of functioning.

Dissociative amnesia

A. The predominant disturbance consists of one or more episodes of an inability to recall important personal information, usually of a traumatic or stressful nature, that is too extensive to be explained by ordinary forgetfulness.
B. The disturbance does not occur exclusively during the course of dissociative identity disorder, dissociative fugue, posttraumatic stress disorder, acute stress disorder, or somatization disorder and is not due to the direct physiologic effects of a substance (such as a drug of abuse or a medication) or a neurologic or other general medical condition (for example, amnestic disorder due to head trauma).
C. The symptoms cause clinically significant distress or impairment in social, occupational, or other important areas of functioning.

Depersonalization disorder

A. The person has persistent or recurring feelings of detachment from, and as if one is an outside observer of, one's mental processes or body (for example, feeling as if one is in a dream).
B. During the depersonalization experience, reality testing remains intact.
C. The depersonalization causes clinically significant distress or impairment in social, occupational, or other important areas of functioning.
D. The depersonalization experience does not occur exclusively during the course of another mental disorder, such as schizophrenia, panic disorder, acute stress disorder, or another dissociative disorder, and is not due to the direct physiologic effects of a substance (such as a drug of abuse or a medication) or a general medical condition (such as temporal lobe epilepsy).

Adapted from *Diagnostic and Statistical Manual of Mental Disorders,* 4th ed., text revision. Washington, D.C.: American Psychiatric Association, 2000 with permission of the publisher.

- ◆ Individual psychodynamic psychotherapy
- ◆ Hypnosis (judicious and circumspect use)
- ◆ Ancillary treatment modalities
  - ◗ Structured formats of art, movement, music, and occupational therapy
  - ◗ Structured groups, conducted by professionals, focusing on the here and now
  - ◗ Supportive family therapy with current significant others (family therapy with families of origin is rarely helpful)
  - ◗ Behavioral interventions (to modify dysfunctional interpersonal interactions)
  - ◗ Cognitive therapy (to strengthen ego functioning and reality testing)
- ◆ Drug therapy (to relieve associated anxiety and depression)
- ◆ Inpatient admission (may be necessary when the patient's safety or the safety of others is at risk)
- ■ Selected nursing diagnoses
  - ◆ Ineffective coping related to inability to deal with multiple personalities
  - ◆ Risk for injury related to suicidal or homicidal impulses
  - ◆ Posttrauma syndrome related to childhood abuse or trauma
- ■ General nursing interventions
  - ◆ Maintain a safe environment; take all necessary safety precautions to protect the patient, other patients, and staff during periods of acting out
  - ◆ Educate unit personnel about the course and treatment of this disorder
  - ◆ Carefully evaluate any participation in the treatment plan by family members (severely dysfunctional families are typically involved in the cause of this disorder)
  - ◆ Administer medications as ordered, and evaluate their effectiveness
  - ◆ Observe and document any personalities that emerge and any precursors to their emergence

❖ Dissociative fugue
- ■ Characteristics
  - ◆ Sudden, unexpected (though apparently purposeful) travel away from home or work, followed by an inability to recall one's past
  - ◆ Confusion about identity, or assumption of a new identity
  - ◆ Severe personal or environmental stress (such as a natural disaster or a war) preceding the psychogenic fugue
  - ◆ Spontaneous, rapid recovery is common
  - ◆ Return to prefugue state may include amnesia for traumatic events, psychological distress, and suicidal and aggressive impulses
- ■ Criteria for medical diagnosis (see the diagnostic criteria for dissociative fugue, page 123.)

- Selected nursing diagnoses
  - ◆ Ineffective coping related to memory loss
  - ◆ Risk for injury related to disorientation
  - ◆ Disturbed personal identity related to loss of old identity and adoption of new one
- Treatment
  - ◆ Thorough investigation of underlying stressors
  - ◆ Psychotherapy (if necessary)
- General nursing interventions
  - ◆ Maintain a safe environment during the fugue state
  - ◆ Reorient the patient to time, place, and person during recovery
  - ◆ Involve the patient's support systems in identifying predisposing stressors
  - ◆ Arrange opportunities for the patient to discuss precipitating factors and feelings about having experienced this disorder, using one-on-one nurse-patient interactions, support groups, or ongoing psychotherapy

❖ Dissociative amnesia
- Characteristics
  - ◆ Sudden memory loss of important personal information
    - ▶ The memory loss is more significant than simple forgetfulness
    - ▶ The memory loss isn't attributable to an organic mental disorder
  - ◆ Memory gaps are usually related to traumatic or extremely stressful events
  - ◆ The events for which there are memory gaps may have lasted from minutes to years
  - ◆ Acute amnesia may resolve spontaneously; individuals with chronic amnesia may gradually begin to recall information
- Types
  - ◆ *Localized amnesia:* inability to remember events that occurred during a circumscribed time, usually after a severely traumatic incident (the most common type)
  - ◆ *Selective amnesia:* inability to remember some of the events that occurred during a circumscribed time
  - ◆ *Generalized amnesia:* inability to remember anything about one's life
  - ◆ *Continuous amnesia:* inability to recall any events that occurred after a specific time, up to and including the present
  - ◆ *Systematized amnesia:* inability to remember certain categories of information
- Criteria for medical diagnosis (see the diagnostic criteria for dissociative amnesia, page 123.)
- Treatment
  - ◆ Supportive care during the amnesia episode
  - ◆ Education regarding the adaptive nature of amnesia symptoms and the need to be cautious and deliberate in overcoming them

◆ Psychotherapy for trauma involves three phases
  ▶ Achieving safety and stability
  ▶ Processing traumatic material (if indicated)
  ▶ Achieving resolution and reintegration (reconnecting with "ordinary life")
■ Selected nursing diagnoses
  ◆ Ineffective coping related to memory loss
  ◆ Risk for injury related to confusion and wandering
  ◆ Disturbed personal identity related to inability to recall the past
■ General nursing interventions
  ◆ Maintain a safe environment during the amnesia episode
  ◆ Reorient the patient to reality as needed
  ◆ Offer opportunities for the patient to discuss precipitating events
  ◆ Provide support for the patient and significant others during recovery

❖ **Depersonalization disorder**
  ■ Characteristics
    ◆ Persistent or recurrent and distressing alteration in perception of one's sense of self such that one's sense of reality is temporarily lost or changed
    ◆ Feelings of detachment (as if an outside observer of oneself) or of being in a mechanical or dreamlike state
    ◆ Various types of sensory anesthesia, lack of affective response, and feelings of not being in control of one's actions
    ◆ Associated features
      ▶ Derealization (a sense that the world is strange or unreal)
      ▶ Alteration in one's perception of surroundings
      ▶ Sense that people are unfamiliar or mechanical
      ▶ Obsessive ruminations
      ▶ Depression
      ▶ Anxiety
      ▶ Somatic complaints
      ▶ Fear of going insane
      ▶ Disturbances in time
    ◆ Intact reality testing
    ◆ Sudden development following exposure to trauma (course may become chronic)
  ■ Criteria for medical diagnosis (see the diagnostic criteria for depersonalization disorder, page 123)
  ■ Treatment
    ◆ Psychotherapy to address issues of control and identity
    ◆ Antidepressant or antianxiety medications
  ■ Selected nursing diagnoses
    ◆ Anxiety related to feelings of lost perception
    ◆ Ineffective coping related to fear of going insane
    ◆ Disturbed self-esteem related to inability to deal with events

◆ Disturbed sensory perception (visual, auditory, kinesthetic, gustatory, tactile, olfactory) related to sensory anesthesia
■ General nursing interventions
◆ Engage the patient in a supportive, one-on-one relationship to alleviate anxiety and worry
◆ Help the patient identify any stressors that may have precipitated the incident
◆ Assist the patient in identifying and developing more effective ways of coping with stress
◆ Teach the patient when to administer medications prescribed for anxiety or depression
◆ Assist the patient in achieving effective reality testing and in maintaining a sense of self; encourage self-care and the expression of perceptions and feelings about the current situation

❖ **Dissociative disorders not otherwise specified**
■ These disorders have a predominant dissociative symptom but don't meet the specific criteria of any single dissociative disorder
■ Treatment, selected nursing diagnoses, and general nursing interventions are similar to those for other dissociative disorders

Clinical situation

Sue Parker, an 18-year-old college freshman, arrives at the University Health Center and asks for a mental health consultation. She reports, hesitantly but with great anxiety, that in the 3 months since college began, she has increasingly begun to feel as if she were unreal, in a dream, that "this couldn't really be me." She reports feeling "like a robot, just going through the motions." She's uncomfortable with these feelings. The latest and most frightening symptom was her sudden awareness that she could no longer "perceive colors." She thinks that she can look at something and identify that it has a color but that she's seeing everything in shades of gray. Sue is worried that she's "going crazy." She says she's doing well at school and making friends.

Sue recently had her college-sports physical examination and was found to have no health problems. A psychosocial assessment reveals that this is Sue's first time away from home and that, 4 months before she began college, her older brother was killed in an auto accident. The doctor's preliminary diagnosis is depersonalization disorder.

Assessment (nursing behaviors and rationales)

1. Perform a health assessment and physical examination. *Physical problems must always be considered as a precipitant or cause of an apparent emotional problem. A thorough physical assessment and review of health history reveal any such problems.*

2. Perform a psychosocial assessment. *A psychosocial assessment helps determine precipitating factors and the degree of impairment.*

3. Assess Sue's perception of the current problem. *The patient's perceptions are the starting point for the nursing intervention. In this case, the patient thought she was "going crazy," not connecting her symptoms with her two recent and significant losses (her brother's death and her absence from home). A nursing assessment brings out this knowledge deficit.*

Nursing diagnoses

- Anxiety related to the frightening symptoms
- Deficient knowledge related to inability to connect recent losses with stress and symptom formation
- Dysfunctional grieving related to leaving home and death of brother
- Disturbed personal identity related to feelings of being unreal
- Disturbed sensory perception (visual) related to inability to perceive color

Planning and goals

- Sue Parker will be treated as an outpatient at the health center.
- She'll experience reduced anxiety so that she can continue in her role performance and engage in psychotherapy.
- She'll begin the healthy grieving process and learn effective coping skills.

Implementation (nursing behaviors and rationales)

1. Engage Sue in a therapeutic relationship. *This is the mechanism for achieving the goals related to anxiety reduction and achievement of healthy coping skills.*
2. Teach Sue about the connection between severe stress levels and the development of psychological symptoms. *By making the patient aware that her severe losses may be an understandable precipitant to her feelings, she may feel less "crazy," stigmatized, and anxious.*
3. Encourage Sue to identify stressors and to develop healthy coping skills. *When the patient is able to see the symptoms as one potential outcome of her dysfunctional grieving, she'll be less anxious and better able to be involved in her own care.*
4. Encourage Sue to continue to participate actively in campus life. *Such participation enables the patient to develop new support systems while strengthening old ones.*

Evaluation

- Sue was able to finish her freshman year and improve her social life as she gradually felt "real" again.
- She became aware that the anniversary of her brother's death (toward the end of the semester) would be a stressful time; she made use of her newly strengthened support systems by expressing her feelings about his death.

Review questions

1. Dissociative identity disorder is characterized by:

   ○ **A.** sudden disruption in consciousness, memory, identity, or perception.

   ○ **B.** sudden memory loss of important personal information.

   ○ **C.** confusion about identity, or assumption of a new identity.

   ○ **D.** chronic posttraumatic stress disorder due to childhood abuse.

   Correct answer: A   Dissociative identity disorder is a sudden disruption in consciousness, memory, identity, and perception involving two or more distinct personality states. Sudden memory loss of important personal information characterizes dissociative amnesia. Confusion about identity or assumption of a new identity are characteristics of dissociative fugue. Individuals who experience chronic posttraumatic stress disorder don't have two or more distinct personality states.

2. The primary treatment for dissociative identity disorder is:

   ○ **A.** hypnosis.

   ○ **B.** individual psychodynamic psychotherapy.

   ○ **C.** family therapy that includes family of origin.

   ○ **D.** group psychotherapy that focuses on early family issues.

   Correct answer: B   Individual psychodynamic psychotherapy is the primary treatment for persons with dissociative identity disorder. Hypnosis may be beneficial, but it should be used judiciously and only by clinicians trained in its use. Therapy that includes the family of origin usually isn't helpful because such families may be severely dysfunctional. Group therapy may be useful, but only if it's structured and focused on the here and now.

3. What are the five types of dissociative amnesia?

   ○ **A.** Localized, selective, generalized, traumatic, circumscribed

   ○ **B.** Localized, selective, generalized, continuous, systematized

   ○ **C.** Localized, selective, acute, chronic, delayed recall

   ○ **D.** Localized, selective, generalized, continuous, complex

   Correct answer: B   Localized, selective, generalized, continuous, and systematized are the five types of dissociative amnesia outlined in *DSM-IV-TR*. Traumatic, circumscribed, acute, chronic, delayed recall, and complex aren't terms used to describe amnesia.

4. What isn't an associated feature of depersonalization disorder?

   ○ **A.** Anxiety and depression

   ○ **B.** Psychotic episodes

   ○ **C.** Somatic complaints

   ○ **D.** Time disturbances

   Correct answer: B Features of depersonalization disorder include anxiety, depression, somatic complaints, and time disturbances. Psychotic episodes aren't an associated feature of depersonalization disorder.

5. What are the three stages of trauma treatment?

   ○ **A.** Achieving safety and security; exploring traumatic material; resolving trauma, abreaction, consolidation of memories

   ○ **B.** Providing support and reassurance, restoring optimal functioning, providing a sense of closure

   ○ **C.** Providing opportunities to discuss the trauma, enhancing memory regarding the trauma, achieving a reduction in trauma symptoms

   ○ **D.** Achieving safety and security, exploring traumatic material, achieving reintegration and resolution

   Correct answer: D Trauma treatment is considered a phasic process, in which safety and stability are emphasized before traumatic material is explored. In the third phase, persons experience previously dissociated material as a part of their life narrative with a decrease in involuntary intrusions, thereby being free to invest energy in other life tasks, such as work, recreation, and relationships.

CHAPTER

13

Mood disorders

❖ Overview
  ■ Mood disorders, also known as affective disorders, are associated with a group of symptoms that result in severe and painful sadness or abnormal elation known clinically as a "high"
  ■ These symptoms change a person's behavior, cognition, motivation, and emotions; in short, they change a person's physical, mental, and social being
  ■ Mood disorders fall into one of two diagnostic categories
    ◆ In *major depressive disorder,* a person experiences one or more episodes of depression with no manic or hypomanic episode
      ❚ The disorder affects twice as many women as men
      ❚ Onset usually occurs in the person's mid-30s
    ◆ In *bipolar I and II mood disorders,* a person experiences major depression with one or more manic or hypomanic episodes
      ❚ Bipolar disorders affect about the same number of men as women
      ❚ Onset usually occurs in the person's late 20s
      ❚ Bipolar disorders have a high prevalence among professional, well-educated groups
      ❚ Approximately 10% of those diagnosed with depression have a bipolar disorder
  ■ Mood disorders vary in frequency, intensity, and duration
  ■ Mood disorders constitute the most common psychiatric diagnosis; about 5% of people in the United States will have a mood disorder; 25% of people with depression have a family member with a mood disorder; 50% of people with bipolar disorder have a family member with a mood disorder

❖ **Major depressive disorder**
  ■ Characteristics
    ◆ Anhedonia
    ◆ Sleep disturbances
    ◆ Loss of libido, appetite, energy, and interest
    ◆ Possible weight loss, fatigue, reduced cognition, and psychomotor agitation
    ◆ Depression that may recur or consist of a single episode
    ◆ Varied degree and intensity of symptoms

- Types
  - ◆ *Agitated depression:* characterized by increased psychomotor activity
  - ◆ *Anxious depression:* characterized by prominent patterns of anxiety
  - ◆ *Atypical depression:* usually involves another condition, such as schizophrenia or dysthymic episode, besides the symptoms of depression
  - ◆ *Chronic depression:* lasts longer than 2 years; about 10% of those diagnosed with depression fall into this category
  - ◆ *Endogenous depression:* characterized by a biological cause, without known external stressors
  - ◆ *Involutional depression:* occurs in the person's late 40s and 50s; women are more prone to involutional depression than are men
  - ◆ *Masked depression:* usually revealed during treatment of somatic complaints
  - ◆ *Paranoid depression:* characterized by paranoid ideation
  - ◆ *Postpartum depression:* can occur after childbirth, in three stages
    - ▶ Within the first 3 to 4 days after delivery, the patient may begin to feel "blue" and sad
    - ▶ About the 3rd week after delivery, other symptoms of depression appear; these symptoms can last for about 1 year
    - ▶ About 3 months after delivery, confusion and disturbances in thought processes begin to accompany other symptoms
  - ◆ *Psychotic depression:* characterized by hallucinations or delusions
  - ◆ *Reactive depression:* associated with external stressors
  - ◆ *Retarded depression:* accompanied by decreased psychomotor activities
  - ◆ *Seasonal depression:* occurs during a specific season of the year
  - ◆ *Drug-induced depression:* results from patient's use of prescription, over-the-counter, or other type of drugs
- Theoretical perspectives
  - ◆ Biochemical theory
    - ▶ Genetic markers have been found that substantiate a hereditary factor
    - ▶ The blood levels of the biogenic amines norepinephrine, dopamine, and serotonin are deficient in people with depression
  - ◆ Psychodynamic theory
    - ▶ Depression results from unresolved grieving in an early stage of the child-parent relationship
    - ▶ The person remains fixed in the anger stage and turns the anger inward, toward the self, resulting in a weak ego and punitive superego
  - ◆ Interpersonal theory
    - ▶ The person is abandoned by or otherwise separated from the parent early in infancy (within the first 6 months), causing incomplete bonding, a predisposing factor
    - ▶ Traumatic separation from a significant other in adulthood can be a precipitating factor; the person then withdraws from family and social contacts

◆ Behavioral theory
  ❒ Depression is believed to result from the interaction of the person-environment-behavior engagement
  ❒ The person has control over personal behavior but not over all environmental influences; consequently, the person may control some aspects of life but not be completely free to choose what happens in life
■ Diagnostic tests
  ◆ Dexamethasone-suppression test: may be useful in diagnosing major depression
    ❒ In a nondepressed person, dexamethasone suppresses the production and release of cortisol from the adrenal gland
    ❒ In a depressed person, this suppression may be only partial or the person may recover more rapidly from the dexamethasone effects
  ◆ Thyrotropin-releasing hormone test: evaluates the ability of the pituitary to produce thyrotropin (decreased thyroid hormone can cause depression)
■ Criteria for medical diagnosis (see the diagnostic criteria for a major depressive episode, page 134)
■ Selected nursing diagnoses
  ◆ Risk for self-directed violence related to low self-esteem
  ◆ Ineffective coping related to guilt feelings
  ◆ Spiritual distress related to feelings of utter despair
  ◆ Disturbed sleep pattern related to desire to escape
  ◆ Impaired verbal communication related to lack of interest
  ◆ Impaired social interaction
■ General nursing interventions
  ◆ Identify the patient's potential for suicide
  ◆ Reevaluate the patient's potential for suicide with any change in mood or behavior
  ◆ Create a safe environment
  ◆ Formulate a verbal contract with the patient to notify staff members when feelings begin to get out of control
  ◆ Encourage the patient to express anger in acceptable ways that are comfortable for the patient
  ◆ Assist the patient in recognizing strengths and accomplishments
  ◆ Teach effective communication skills
  ◆ Assist the patient in performing activities of daily living (ADLs)
  ◆ Provide positive reinforcement of acceptable behaviors
  ◆ Assist the patient in setting realistic goals
  ◆ Help the patient clarify thought processes
  ◆ Discourage sleeping other than at bedtime
  ◆ Teach relaxation techniques to use before bedtime
  ◆ Limit time spent alone by encouraging participation in group activities
  ◆ Provide simple activities that the patient can successfully complete

(Text continues on page 137.)

Diagnostic criteria for mood disorders

Here are the *DSM-IV-TR* diagnostic criteria for the mood disorders discussed in this chapter.

Major depressive episode

A. Five or more of the following symptoms have been present during the same 2 weeks and represent a change from previous functioning; at least one of the symptoms is either (1) depressed mood or (2) loss of interest or pleasure. *Note:* Do not include symptoms that are clearly due to a general medical condition or mood-incongruent delusions or hallucinations.
  1. Depressed mood most of the day, nearly every day, as indicated by subjective report (for example, feels sad or empty) or observation made by others (for example, appears tearful). *Note:* in children and adolescents, the indicator can be irritable mood.
  2. Markedly diminished interest or pleasure in all, or almost all, daily activities nearly every day (as indicated by subjective account or observation made by others)
  3. Significant weight loss when not dieting, weight gain (such as a change of more than 5% in body weight in 1 month), or a decrease or increase in appetite, nearly every day. *Note:* In children, consider failure to make expected weight gains.
  4. Insomnia or hypersomnia nearly every day
  5. Psychomotor agitation or retardation nearly every day (observable by others, not merely subjective feelings of restlessness or being slowed down)
  6. Fatigue or loss of energy nearly every day
  7. Feelings of worthlessness or excessive or inappropriate guilt (which may be delusional) nearly every day (not merely self-reproach or guilt about being sick)
  8. Diminished ability to think or concentrate, or indecisiveness, nearly every day (either by subjective account or as observed by others)
  9. Recurrent thoughts of death (not just fear of dying), recurrent suicidal ideation without a specific plan, or a suicide attempt or a specific plan for committing suicide
B. The symptoms do not meet criteria for a mixed episode.
C. The symptoms cause clinically significant distress or impairment in social, occupational, or other important areas of functioning.
D. The symptoms are not due to the direct physiologic effects of a substance (such as a drug of abuse or a medication) or a general medical condition (such as hypothyroidism).
E. The symptoms are not better accounted for by bereavement (after the loss of a loved one, symptoms persist for longer than 2 months or are characterized by marked functional impairment, morbid preoccupation with worthlessness, suicidal ideation, psychotic symptoms, or psychomotor retardation).

Manic episode

A. The person experiences a distinct period of abnormality and persistently elevated, expansive, or irritable mood, lasting at least 1 week (or any duration if hospitalization is necessary).
B. During the period of mood disturbance, three or more of the following symptoms have persisted (four if the mood is only irritable) and have been present to a significant degree:
  1. Inflated self-esteem or grandiosity
  2. Decreased need for sleep (for example, feels rested after only 3 hours of sleep)
  3. Unusual talkativeness or pressure to keep talking
  4. Flight of ideas or subjective experience that thoughts are racing
  5. Distractibility (attention too easily drawn to unimportant or irrelevant external stimuli)
  6. Increase in goal-directed activity (either socially, at work or school, or sexually) or psychomotor agitation
  7. Excessive involvement in pleasurable activities that have a high potential for painful consequences (engaging in unrestrained buying sprees, sexual indiscretions, or foolish business investments)
C. The symptoms do not meet criteria for a mixed episode.
D. The mood disturbance is sufficiently severe to cause marked impairment in occupational functioning or in usual social activities or relationships with others or to necessitate hospitalization to prevent harm to self or others, or the patient exhibits psychotic features.
E. The symptoms are not due to the direct physiologic effects of a substance (such as a drug of abuse, a medication, or other treatment) or a general medical condition (such as hyperthyroidism).

Diagnostic criteria for mood disorders *(continued)*

Note: Maniclike episodes that are clearly caused by somatic antidepressant treatment (medication, electroconvulsive therapy, light therapy) should not count toward a diagnosis of Bipolar I disorder.

Bipolar I disorder, single manic episode

A. The person experiences only one manic episode and has no past major depressive episodes.
Note: Recurrence is defined as either a change in polarity from depression or an interval of at least 2 months without manic symptoms.
B. The manic episode isn't better accounted for by schizoaffective disorder and isn't superimposed on schizophrenia, schizophreniform disorder, delusional disorder, or psychotic disorder not otherwise specified.
Specify if:
Mixed: if symptoms meet criteria for a mixed episode.
Specify (for current or most recent episode):
Severity/Psychotic/Remission Specifiers
With Catatonic Features
With Postpartum Onset

Bipolar I disorder, most recent episode hypomanic

A. The person is currently (or most recently) in a hypomanic episode.
B. The person has previously experienced at least one manic episode or mixed episode.
C. The mood symptoms cause clinically significant distress or impairment in social, occupational, or other important areas of functioning.
D. The mood episodes in criteria A and B are not better accounted for by schizoaffective disorder and are not superimposed on schizophrenia, schizophreniform disorder, delusional disorder, or psychotic disorder not otherwise specified.
Specify if:
Longitudinal Course Specifiers (With and Without Interepisode Recovery)
With Seasonal Pattern
With Rapid Cycling

Bipolar I disorder, most recent episode manic

A. The person is currently (or most recently) in a manic episode.
B. The person has experienced at least one major depressive episode, manic episode, or mixed episode.
C. The mood episodes in criteria A and B are not better accounted for by schizoaffective disorder and are not superimposed on schizophrenia, schizophreniform disorder, delusional disorder, or psychotic disorder not otherwise specified.
Specify (for current or most recent episode):
Severity/Psychotic/Remission Specifiers
With Catatonic Features
With Postpartum Onset
Specify:
Longitudinal Course Specifiers (With and Without Interepisode Recovery)
With Seasonal Pattern (applies only to the pattern of major depressive episodes)
With Rapid Cycling

Bipolar I disorder, most recent episode mixed

A. The person is currently (or most recently) in a mixed episode.
B. The person has experienced at least one major depressive episode, manic episode, or mixed episode.
C. The mood episodes in criteria A and B are not better accounted for by schizoaffective disorder and are not superimposed on schizophrenia, schizophreniform disorder, delusional disorder, or psychotic disorder not otherwise specified.
Specify (for current or most recent episode):

(continued)

Diagnostic criteria for mood disorders *(continued)*

Severity/Psychotic/Remission Specifiers
With Catatonic Features
With Postpartum Onset
Specify:
Longitudinal Course Specifiers (With and Without Interepisode Recovery)
With Seasonal Pattern (applies only to the pattern of major depressive episodes)
With Rapid Cycling

Bipolar II disorder

A. The person has or had one or more major depressive episodes.
B. The person has or had at least one hypomanic episode.
C. The person has never had a manic episode or a mixed episode.
D. The mood symptoms in criteria A and B are not better accounted for by schizoaffective disorder and are not superimposed on schizophrenia, schizophreniform disorder, delusional disorder, or psychotic disorder not otherwise specified.
E. The symptoms cause clinically significant distress or impairment in social, occupational, or other important areas of functioning.
Specify (for current or most recent episode):
Hypomanic: if currently (or most recently) in a hypomanic episode
Depressed: if currently (or most recently) in a major depressive episode
Specify (for current or most recent major depressive episode only if it is the most recent type of mood episode):
Severity/Psychotic/Remission Specifiers
Note: Fifth-digit codes specified cannot be used here because the code for Bipolar II Disorder already uses the fifth digit.
Chronic
With Catatonic Features
With Melancholic Features
With Atypical Features
With Postpartum Onset
Specify:
Longitudinal Course Specifiers (With and Without Interepisode Recovery)
With Seasonal Pattern (applies only to the pattern of major depressive episodes)
With Rapid Cycling

Cyclothymic disorder

A. For at least 2 years, the person has numerous periods with hypomanic symptoms and numerous periods with depressive symptoms that do not meet criteria for a major depressive episode.
Note: In children and adolescents, the duration must be at least 1 year.
B. During the above 2-year period (1 year in children and adolescents), the person hasn't been without the symptoms in criterion A for more than 2 months at a time.
C. No major depressive episode, manic episode, or mixed episode has been present during the first 2 years of the disturbance.
Note: After the initial 2 years (1 year in children and adolescents) of cyclothymic disorder, there may be superimposed manic or mixed episodes (in which case both bipolar I disorder and cyclothymic disorder may be diagnosed) or major depressive episodes (in which case both bipolar II disorder and cyclothymic disorder may be diagnosed).
D. The symptoms in criterion A are not better accounted for by schizoaffective disorder and are not superimposed on schizophrenia, schizophreniform disorder, delusional disorder, or psychotic disorder not otherwise specified.
E. The symptoms are not due to the direct physiologic effects of a substance (such as a drug of abuse or a medication) or a general medical condition (such as hyperthyroidism).
F. The symptoms cause clinically significant distress or impairment in social, occupational, or other important areas of functioning.

Adapted from *Diagnostic and Statistical Manual of Mental Disorders,* 4th ed., text revision. Washington, D.C.: American Psychiatric Association, 2000 with permission of the publisher.

◆ Administer selective serotonin reuptake inhibitors, tricyclic antidepressants, or monoamine oxidase inhibitors as prescribed
◆ Discuss the concepts of loss and grief with the patient
◆ Help the patient identify and eliminate cognitive distortions

❖ Bipolar disorders

■ Characteristics

◆ Symptoms of at least one episode of mania, often accompanied by a major depressive episode
◆ Potential for psychotic features

■ Types

◆ *Bipolar I disorder, manic:* characterized by elation or irritability with excessive motor activity
◆ *Bipolar I disorder, mixed:* characterized by mood swings ranging from depression to euphoria, with intervening periods of normal behavior
◆ *Bipolar II disorder:* characterized by at least one manic episode accompanied by hypomania
◆ *Cyclothymic disorder:* characterized by a chronic, fluctuating mood disturbance with frequent periods of hypomania and depression

■ Theoretical perspectives

◆ Biological theory

▶ Genetic predisposition exists, especially if a female is diagnosed with the condition
▶ Increased levels of norepinephrine, a biogenic amine, appear in the brain of a manic patient

◆ Psychoanalytic theory

▶ Cyclic behaviors of depression and mania are responses to conditional love from the significant caregiver
▶ Ego development is disrupted because the child is in a dependent role, resulting in a punitive superego or a strong id

■ Criteria for medical diagnosis (see the diagnostic criteria for bipolar disorders, pages 135 and 136)

■ Selected nursing diagnoses

◆ Risk for injury related to agitation
◆ Ineffective health maintenance related to hyperactivity
◆ Disturbed sleep pattern related to restlessness
◆ Dressing or grooming self-care deficit related to inattention to personal needs
◆ Impaired social interaction related to decreased attention span
◆ Disturbed thought processes related to the psychotic process
◆ Imbalanced nutrition: Less than body requirements related to hyperactivity

■ General nursing interventions

◆ Reduce environmental stimuli
◆ Limit the patient's participation in group activities
◆ Create a safe environment

◆ Provide physical exercise as a substitute for increased motor activity
◆ Avoid arguments or confrontations with the patient
◆ Instruct the patient on using more socially appropriate behaviors
◆ Provide positive feedback for socially acceptable behaviors
◆ Monitor eating and sleeping patterns
◆ Restrict caffeine intake
◆ Limit the selection of clothing available
◆ Set goals for minimal standards of personal hygiene
◆ Keep the patient oriented to reality
◆ Assist the patient in focusing on a single task
◆ Limit invasion of the patient's personal space by other patients and staff
◆ Encourage rest periods
◆ Administer lithium, antianxiety agents, or antipsychotics as prescribed

Clinical situation

Mary Boggs, age 36, is admitted to the inpatient psychiatric treatment facility of a local hospital with a tentative diagnosis of major depressive disorder. She has just been treated in the emergency department for attempting suicide by taking 20 tablets of Xanax 10 mg. About 3 months ago, Mary's boyfriend broke off his relationship with her to pursue another woman. Since that time, Mary has been put on probation at work because of many absences and her inability to complete work assignments.

Mary states that she has trouble sleeping and hasn't been able to concentrate. Finding no humor in life, she dreads getting out of bed in the morning to face the world and she has stopped socializing with her girlfriends. Mary says she has never felt this bad before and can't seem to get her life together. She feels worthless; she apologizes to you for her lack of personal hygiene, saying that she was never like this before.

Mary states that she had lived with her boyfriend for 6 years; when they broke up, she had to move back home because of inadequate finances. Since then, her parents have told her that she'll never amount to anything.

Assessment (nursing behaviors and rationales)

1. Perform a physical assessment, noting any somatic complaints, changes in eating and sleeping patterns, and level of concentration. *Physical problems (such as tumors, infections, endocrine disorders, anemia, and electrolyte imbalances) can produce depressive symptoms.*

2. Assess whether Mary can meet self-care needs satisfactorily. *Performing ADLs may be difficult for a depressed person, whose energy level typically decreases. Failure to meet self-care needs leads to feelings of hopelessness and unworthiness.*

3. Assess Mary's potential for suicide; determine whether she's currently suicidal. *Patients with a history of suicide attempts and those who are depressed* *are at higher risk for attempting suicide than patients with no history or depressive symptoms. Patients whose depression is lifting are at higher risk of suicide than those severely depressed because they now have the energy, as the depression lifts, to commit suicide.*

4. Perform a psychosocial assessment, inquiring about social interaction and coping patterns, life stressors, and previous experiences with sadness. *Having the patient explain previous behaviors assists the nurse in determining the severity and duration of the current depression.*

5. Assess Mary's perception of the situation. *Distorted perceptions about what's happening is a symptom of depression. Changes in perceptions suggest changes in the depressed state.*

Nursing diagnoses

- Risk for self-directed violence related to despair
- Ineffective coping related to anxiety
- Chronic low self-esteem related to feelings of worthlessness
- Social isolation related to withdrawn behavior
- Disturbed sleep pattern related to worrying

Planning and goals

- Mary Boggs will remain safe from suicidal impulses.
- She'll express thoughts and feelings about her loss.
- She'll perform ADLs, such as personal hygiene, independently.
- She'll speak positively about her appearance and accomplishments.
- She'll be able to sleep at least 6 hours nightly by the time of discharge.

Implementation (nursing behaviors and rationales)

1. Monitor Mary's potential for suicide by directly asking her whether she's suicidal. *Patients who have attempted suicide are at higher risk than those who haven't. Most people who state an intention to commit suicide ultimately succeed unless someone intervenes. Psychotic thoughts add to the suicide risk.*

2. Place Mary on suicidal observation, if indicated. Explain that you want to keep her safe until she can keep herself safe. *In an unsafe environment, suicidal people are more likely to attempt suicide impulsively. The nurse's caring attitude may give the patient a sense of protection. Suicide precautions (including monitoring the patient's whereabouts, bathroom use, use of personal-care items, and taking of medication) provide safety for the patient.*

3. Secure a promise from Mary that she'll talk to a staff member if suicidal thoughts emerge. *Suicidal patients require a safe, secure environment, along with staff members who will be there to prevent a suicide attempt, if necessary. Having someone to talk with may reduce the patient's anxiety.*

4. Encourage Mary to verbalize her feelings about her previous romantic relationship. *Talking about these feelings may help the patient begin to deal more effectively with the loss.*

5. Have Mary describe what happened at work and home before she came to the hospital. *This helps the patient see her problems from a different perspec-*

tive. *By learning to consider all aspects of a situation, the patient is developing an effective coping strategy.*

6. Help Mary develop goals, resources, and coping skills for handling her grief. *Developing realistic goals and identifying resources promotes independence and self-esteem and assists the patient in positively handling her grief. Strengthening coping skills enhances her ability to grieve successfully.*

7. Promote the development of Mary's social and leisure skills. *This helps the patient regain self-confidence and assists in reducing her social isolation.*

8. Involve Mary in physical exercise and play activities. *These activities release tension and promote the development of new coping skills.*

9. Assist Mary in identifying people she can ask for help after being discharged. *Having a support system decreases feelings of despair and reduces the likelihood of future suicide attempts.*

10. Teach Mary and her family about depressive behavior. *The patient and her family probably don't understand that her behavior is the result of an illness. Knowledge about depression helps the patient deal more effectively with her behavior and enables her family to be more supportive during her postdischarge treatment.*

Evaluation

- Mary makes no further attempts at suicide.
- She attends to her ADLs without assistance.
- She sleeps a minimum of 6 hours at night.
- She participates in social activities with other patients and staff.
- She sets realistic goals for her work and living arrangements.
- She develops a support system of family and friends.

Review questions

1. The nurse collaborates with a patient to develop goals to increase the patient's self-esteem. When working with this patient, the nurse should keep in mind that depressed patients commonly:

○ **A.** set goals that require minimal effort on their part.

○ **B.** have little desire to change the status quo.

○ **C.** overestimate their abilities and skills.

○ **D.** set up problems by establishing unrealistic goals.

Correct answer: D Depressed patients commonly set unattainable goals for themselves because they tend to think in "all-or-nothing" terms. These patients require help in breaking down major goals into smaller, more manageable goals that can be realistically accomplished.

2. Which nurse's note best describes the appearance of a depressed person?

○ **A.** "Sat in chair, not talking to anyone, seems unaware of surroundings"

○ **B.** "Apparently very depressed and withdrawn, not communicating with anyone"

○ **C.** "Sat with hands in lap, gazing at floor, didn't speak to others"

○ **D.** "Appeared sad and lonely, not communicating with other patients"

Correct answer: C   Nurse's notes should describe the actual behaviors of the depressed patient. Depressed patients are commonly socially withdrawn and noncommunicative, and they tend to avoid eye contact. The remaining options contain subjective observations by the nurse.

3. A 50-year-old man is depressed and has been in bed most of the day. What's the best action for the nurse to take at mealtime?

○ **A.** Take him to the dining room and sit with him as he eats.

○ **B.** Ask him when, where, and what he prefers to eat.

○ **C.** Give him a tray with finger foods in his room.

○ **D.** Encourage him to eat, and explain the importance of nutrition.

Correct answer: A   The best action is to help the client meet his nutritional needs by taking him to the dining area. By staying with the patient during the meal, the nurse can encourage both eating and socializing. The remaining options don't encourage socialization with others.

4. A patient with bipolar disorder is disruptive in group and social settings. What intervention could the nurse implement to assist the patient in developing social skills?

○ **A.** Encourage support with self-care.

○ **B.** Assist in decreasing the patient's activity level.

○ **C.** Facilitate one-to-one opportunities.

○ **D.** Establish guidelines for behavior.

Correct answer: D   The patient must be helped to set limits and establish guidelines for appropriate behavior. Bipolar patients have the tendency to put their needs first and violate the rights of others. Options A, B, and C don't address this behavioral issue.

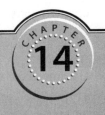

Delirium, dementia, and amnestic disorders

❖ **Overview**
- The primary disturbance in delirium, dementia, and amnestic disorders is a manifest and substantive deficit in memory or cognition that significantly changes a person's level of functioning
- A medical condition (not always readily identifiable) and substance abuse are the two primary causes
- Formerly known as organic mental disorders, these conditions were renamed in *DSM-IV-TR* because of an incorrect implication that other mental disorders don't have an organic cause
- Specific medical conditions can further differentiate the diagnosis

❖ **Delirium**
- Characteristics
  - ◆ Acute brain dysfunction marked by a deficiency in the capacity to maintain attention
  - ◆ Result of various physical causes, including infection, an endocrine disorder, trauma, and drug abuse
  - ◆ Rapid onset (within hours or days) and usually brief duration
  - ◆ Varying course of illness that depends on identifying and correcting the causative agent
- Signs and symptoms
  - ◆ Disorganized thought processes
  - ◆ Apathy
  - ◆ Clouded sensorium
  - ◆ Impaired cognition
  - ◆ Decreased level of consciousness
  - ◆ Disorientation
  - ◆ Disturbances in perception
- Criteria for medical diagnosis (see the diagnostic criteria for delirium)
- Selected nursing diagnoses
  - ◆ Disturbed thought processes related to changes in brain function
  - ◆ Impaired verbal communication related to incoherent speech
  - ◆ Dressing or grooming self-care deficit related to inability to perform activities of daily living (ADLs)
  - ◆ Disturbed sensory perception (visual) related to disorientation

Diagnostic criteria for delirium, dementia, and amnestic disorders

Here are the *DSM-IV-TR* diagnostic criteria for delirium, dementia, and amnestic disorders.

Delirium

A. The person has a reduced ability to maintain attention to external stimuli (for example, questions must be repeated because the person's attention wanders) and to shift attention appropriately to new external stimuli (for example, the person continues to repeat the answer to a previous question).

B. The person exhibits disorganized thinking, as indicated by rambling, irrelevant, or incoherent speech.

C. The person experiences at least two of the following:
   1. Reduced level of consciousness (such as difficulty keeping awake during the examination)
   2. Perceptual disturbances: misinterpretations, illusions, or hallucinations
   3. Disturbance of sleep-wake cycle with insomnia or daytime sleepiness
   4. Increased or decreased psychomotor activity
   5. Disorientation to time, place, or person
   6. Memory impairment (for instance, an inability to learn new material, such as the names of several unrelated objects after 5 minutes, or to remember past events, such as the history of the current episode of illness)

D. Clinical features develop over a short period (usually hours to days) and tend to fluctuate over the course of the day.

E. The disturbance meets either of the following criteria:
   1. The history, physical examination, or laboratory tests show evidence of one or more specific organic factors judged to be etiologically related to the disturbance.
   2. The disturbance cannot be accounted for by any nonorganic mental disorder (such as a manic episode accounting for agitation and sleep disturbance).

Dementia

A. The person shows demonstrable evidence of short- and long-term memory impairment.
   1. Short-term memory impairment (inability to learn new information) may be indicated by an inability to remember three objects after 5 minutes.
   2. Long-term memory impairment (inability to remember information previously known) may be indicated by an inability to remember personal information (such as one's birthplace or occupation) or facts of common knowledge (such as past U.S. presidents or well-known historical dates).

B. The person exhibits at least one of the following:
   1. Impairment in abstract thinking, as indicated by an inability to find similarities and differences between related words, difficulty in defining words and concepts, and other similar tasks
   2. Impaired judgment, as indicated by an inability to make reasonable plans to deal with interpersonal, family, and job-related problems and issues
   3. Other disturbances of higher cortical function, such as aphasia (disorder of language), apraxia (inability to carry out motor activities despite intact comprehension and motor function), agnosia (failure to recognize or identify objects despite intact sensory function), and "constructional difficulty" (for example, an inability to copy three-dimensional figures, assemble blocks, or arrange sticks in specific designs)
   4. Personality change (that is, an alteration or accentuation of premorbid traits)

C. The disturbance in A and B significantly interferes with the person's work or usual social activities or relationships with others.

D. The disturbance does not occur exclusively during the course of delirium.

E. The disturbance meets either of the following criteria:
   1. The history, physical examination, or laboratory tests show evidence of one or more specific organic factors judged to be etiologically related to the disturbance.
   2. The disturbance cannot be accounted for by any nonorganic mental disorder (such as major depression accounting for cognitive impairment).

Health care professionals use the following criteria to determine the severity of dementia:

Mild: Although work or social activities are significantly impaired, the capacity for independent living remains, with adequate personal hygiene and relatively intact judgment.

Moderate: Independent living is hazardous, and some degree of supervision is necessary.

(continued)

Diagnostic criteria for delirium, dementia, and amnestic disorders *(continued)*

Severe: Activities of daily living are so impaired that continual supervision is required (for instance, the person cannot maintain minimal personal hygiene or is largely incoherent or mute).

Amnestic disorders

A. The person shows demonstrable evidence of short- and long-term memory impairment.
  1. Short-term memory impairment (inability to learn new information) may be indicated by an inability to remember three objects after 5 minutes.
  2. Long-term memory impairment (inability to remember information previously known) may be indicated by an inability to remember personal information (such as one's birthplace or occupation) or facts of common knowledge (such as past U.S. presidents or well-known historical dates); the person remembers extremely remote events better than more recent events.

B. The disturbance does not occur exclusively during the course of delirium and does not meet the criteria for dementia (that is, the person shows no impairment in abstract thinking or judgment, no other disturbances of higher cortical function, and no personality change).

C. The history, physical examination, or laboratory tests show evidence of one or more specific organic factors judged to be etiologically related to the disturbance.

Adapted from *Diagnostic and Statistical Manual of Mental Disorders,* 4th ed., text revision. Washington, D.C.: American Psychiatric Association, 2000 with permission of the publisher.

- General nursing interventions
  - Assist the patient with reality orientation
    - Call the patient by name
    - Keep a clock and calendar in plain view
  - Use simple words and short sentences to communicate
  - Assist the patient with personal hygiene; establish a routine for dressing
  - Provide a safe, quiet environment

- ❖ **Dementia**
  - Characteristics
    - Memory impairment and insidious loss of intellectual ability
    - Onset tends to be gradual (such as from Alzheimer's disease or acquired immunodeficiency syndrome)
    - Progressive, static, or recurring course, depending on pathogenesis
    - Prevalence among elderly patients (but can occur in any age-group)
  - Signs and symptoms
    - Short- and long-term memory impairment
    - Premorbid personality changes
    - Disturbed judgment
    - Difficulty in understanding the meaning of words
    - Confusion
    - Depressed affect
  - Criteria for medical diagnosis (see the diagnostic criteria for dementia, pages 143 and 144)

■ Selected nursing diagnoses
◆ Disturbed thought processes related to inaccurate interpretation of environmental stimuli
◆ Imbalanced nutrition: Less than body requirements related to failure to remember mealtimes
◆ Risk for injury related to disorientation and confusion
◆ Compromised family coping related to family's inability to deal with changes in the patient's personality
■ General nursing interventions
◆ Assist the patient with reality orientation
◆ Label furniture, rooms, and clothing
◆ Speak slowly and repeat instructions several times
◆ Provide a safe environment
◆ Frequently monitor the patient's whereabouts
◆ Put the patient on a consistent meal schedule; observe the patient's food intake
◆ Teach the patient's family about the disease and how they can adjust to changes in the patient's behavior

❖ **Amnestic disorders**
■ Characteristics
◆ Short- and long-term memory impairment without clouding of consciousness or intellectual deterioration
◆ Result of a specific organic insult to the brain
▶ Anterograde memory loss (the patient can't remember events that occurred after the brain insult)
▶ Retrograde memory loss (the patient can't remember events that occurred before the brain insult)
◆ Confabulation commonly used as a defense mechanism
■ Signs and symptoms
◆ Inability to recall recent events
◆ Inability to retain newly learned material
◆ Observable or laboratory test evidence of organic brain insult (such as from trauma or a vitamin deficiency)
■ Criteria for medical diagnosis (see the diagnostic criteria for amnestic disorders)
■ Selected nursing diagnoses
◆ Imbalanced nutrition: Less than body requirements related to a nutrient deficiency
◆ Impaired adjustment related to memory loss
◆ Risk for injury related to inability to learn safety rules
◆ Compromised family coping related to poor family adjustment to the patient's behavior
■ General nursing interventions
◆ Monitor the patient's food and fluid intake
◆ Supervise the patient's travel away from home

◆ Establish a training program for relearning information needed to exist safely in the environment

◆ Institute memory therapy (for example, by teaching mnemonics)

◆ Teach the family coping techniques and ways to meet the patient's safety needs

Clinical situation

Mary Smith, a 65-year-old female, is brought to the emergency department by her spouse. Her husband reports that when he came home from work, he found Mary in a very unusual state of mind. She typically has their supper prepared and is eager to see him, but this evening he found her dozing in a chair. After Mary woke up, she was confused, lethargic, and disoriented to time and place. When her spouse tried to talk with her, she was unable to respond appropriately to his questions. Her answers were mumbled and nonsensical. Her spouse also reports that the previous evening Mary had complained of left flank pain and feeling a little warm. She's admitted to the hospital with the diagnosis of delirium, ruling out urinary tract infection.

Assessment (nursing behaviors and rationales)

1. Perform a physical assessment. Obtain Mary's medical history from her spouse. Note history of kidney disease, urinary tract infections and treatment, history of head trauma, other illnesses, allergies, and medications. *Prior illnesses and disease processes may contribute to the patient's current mental state.*

2. Perform a Mini–Mental Status Examination. Assess Mary's orientation, appropriate responses, affect, memory recall, insight, judgment, psychosis, and thought processes. *This information is invaluable in determining appropriate treatment.*

3. Assess Mary's personality changes and premorbid level of functioning. *Information regarding acute or gradual changes in the patient's personality and functioning may help determine diagnosis and reversal of changed mental status.*

4. Assess Mary's ability to perform self-care. *Confusion and disorientation may reduce the patient's ability to care for herself and perform ADLs independently.*

5. Assess for safety in Mary's new environment. *Confusion and disorientation may cause the patient to injure herself.*

Nursing diagnoses

● Disturbed thought processes related to confusion and disorientation

● Risk for injury related to confusion

● Dressing or grooming self-care deficit related to cognitive impairment

Planning and goals

● Mary will be oriented to reality.

● She'll be provided with assistance in ADLs.

● She'll be maintained in a safe environment.

● She'll return to a premorbid level of mental functioning.

Implementation (nursing behaviors and rationales)

1. Address Mary by her name, use familiar objects to orient her to reality, and provide her with a calendar and a clock. *Calling the patient by name helps retain individuality; familiar objects, calendars, and clocks promote orientation to time and place.*

2. Assist Mary with ADLs as needed. *Helping the patient perform basic hygiene and care measures promotes self-esteem without exhausting her.*

3. Provide frequent rest periods as needed, and promote a nutritious diet. *Frequent rest periods help to conserve the patient's energy, while a diet that provides adequate calories and nutrients helps to meet her nutritional needs.*

4. Assist with safety measures. *Taking steps to ensure safety will prevent injury to the patient and others.*

5. Monitor Mary's laboratory test results, vital signs, intake and output, and response to medications. *Determining the patient's therapeutic response as well as noting adverse effects of medications and therapies will help direct the course of treatment.*

Evaluation

● Mrs. Smith is aware that she's in the hospital, and she's oriented to day, time, and person.
● She responds appropriately in conversation.
● She can perform ADLs independently.
● She has returned to a premorbid level of mental functioning.

Review questions

1. A man is found wandering along the roadside. He's unable to tell the ambulance staff his name, address, or phone number, and he has difficulty articulating his words. His responses don't correspond to the questions asked. He seems to be looking for something and appears lost. His family is contacted, and they report that he has had a progressive deterioration of cognitive functioning over the past year and has wandered off multiple times in the recent past. What diagnosis would correspond with his symptoms?

○ **A.** Dementia

○ **B.** Delirium

○ **C.** Amnesia

○ **D.** Drug abuse

Correct answer: A Dementia presents with a gradual decline in cognitive functioning. Delirium has an acute onset. Amnesia usually follows a trauma or injury, which isn't supported in this patient's situation. The patient doesn't exhibit evidence of drug abuse.

2. A man is diagnosed with dementia. He exhibits confusion, disorientation, wandering behaviors, decreased appetite, and sleep disturbance. What nursing diagnosis is a priority for this patient?

○ **A.** Disturbed thought processes

○ **B.** Imbalanced nutrition: Less than body requirements

○ **C.** Risk for injury

○ **D.** Disturbed sleep pattern

Correct answer: C Safety is a top priority for patients with dementia because they're at high risk for unsafe behaviors and cognitively unaware of potential dangers. The patient's nutritional status, sleep patterns, and altered thought processes will need to be addressed throughout the course of treatment, but they aren't top priorities.

3. A woman's family brings her to the emergency department and reports symptoms of an acute onset of mental status change, including confusion, disorientation, lethargy, and decreased psychomotor activity. What diagnosis corresponds with her symptoms?

○ **A.** Dementia

○ **B.** Amnesia

○ **C.** Delirium

○ **D.** Drug abuse

Correct answer: C The distinguishing symptom of delirium is an acute onset. Dementia tends to have a more gradual onset of symptoms. Amnesia typically follows trauma or injury. A patient who abuses drugs would exhibit signs and symptoms of withdrawal.

4. A man is found unconscious in his car after crashing into a tree. On arrival to the emergency department, he's conscious but has no memory of recent and remote events. His family arrives and provides a medical and psychiatric history. They report that, except for the memory impairment, he appears to be his usual self. Medical tests reveal a concussion. What diagnosis would the nurse expect the man to have?

○ **A.** Dementia

○ **B.** Amnesia

○ **C.** Delirium

○ **D.** Alcohol abuse

Correct answer: B Memory impairment and evidence of one or more specific organic factors related to the disturbance are signs of amnesia. Dementia and delirium are slower in onset than amnesia. The patient doesn't exhibit evidence to support a diagnosis of alcohol abuse.

5. A patient is hospitalized on a dementia unit. He exhibits agitation and restlessness, shouts obscenities, and appears to be hallucinating. Which intervention should the nurse initially implement?

  ○ **A.** Place him in a geri chair.

  ○ **B.** Administer haloperidol lactate (Haldol) 5 mg I.M.

  ○ **C.** Take him to a quiet place.

  ○ **D.** Call him by name and escort him to a quiet area.

Correct answer: D Orienting the patient to reality and escorting him to a quiet area are the most important interventions for a patient with dementia. Geri chairs and I.M. medications are considered restraints.

Personality disorders

❖ Overview
- On a social response continuum, interpersonal relationships range from adaptive behaviors to maladaptive ones
  - ◆ Adaptive behaviors provide for mutually satisfying interactions
  - ◆ Maladaptive behaviors result in loneliness, suspiciousness, and withdrawn behavior
- Personality disorders fall somewhere within the maladaptive range; the degree of maladaptation depends on the type of disorder and the severity of symptoms and is characterized by an enduring pattern of inner experience and behavior that deviates markedly from the cultural norm
- The behavioral responses of a person with a personality disorder are inflexible; onset occurs in adolescence or early adulthood and creates impairment or distress
  - ◆ The behaviors cause marked social impairment and disruption in vocational functioning; in short, they render the person incapable of functioning effectively in society
  - ◆ The person remains unaware of these adverse impacts
  - ◆ The person reacts to stress and anxiety by trying to change the surrounding environment
  - ◆ The person perceives character flaws not only as acceptable and unobjectionable to others but also as positive aspects of his or her character
  - ◆ The person doesn't accept blame for hurting someone
- The *DSM-IV-TR* classifies personality disorders as Axis II diagnoses that fall into one of three clusters based on descriptive commonalities
  - ◆ Cluster A consists of paranoid, schizoid, and schizotypal personality disorders
    - ▶ A person with one of these disorders is aloof and emotionally distant from others
    - ▶ The person's behaviors are considered strange or eccentric
  - ◆ Cluster B consists of antisocial, borderline, histrionic, and narcissistic personality disorders
    - ▶ A person with one of these disorders appears extremely egocentric, with little ability to understand another's perspective
    - ▶ The person's behaviors are erratic and dramatic

◆ Cluster C consists of avoidant, dependent, and obsessive-compulsive personality disorders and those not otherwise specified

> ▶ A person with one of these disorders appears overly anxious about various social and personal issues
>
> ▶ The person tends to be unusually concerned with rules, procedures, and acceptance by others

❖ Theoretical perspectives

■ Biological theory

◆ A genetic predisposition to personality disorders exists, especially among people with a cluster A disorder or those with a family history of alcoholism or another psychiatric problem

◆ A person with schizoid and a personality disorder, for example, is likely to have a family member who is schizophrenic

■ Psychodynamic theory

◆ Poor parenting during the first 5 years of life results in inadequate mastery of developmental issues and conflicts centering on autonomy, separation-individuation, abandonment, dependency, control, or authority

◆ People who have had a cold, indifferent, and emotionally deficient childhood have a good chance of developing a personality disorder

■ Sociocultural theory

◆ In some cultures, gender-specific child-rearing practices may predispose women to dependent personality disorder

◆ Cultural norms influence the establishment of relationships; casual friendships may not be encouraged

◆ Social mobility and lack of close family ties promote loneliness and involuntary isolation

◆ Harsh or abusive parental treatment or abandonment may be a factor for personality disorders

❖ Paranoid personality disorder

■ Characteristics

◆ Suspiciousness

◆ Conviction that other people "are out to do me in"

◆ Inability to discern the context of a given situation, so that the person misperceives single acts or events within the situation

◆ Cold, aloof, overly serious affect

◆ Inability to experience or express warmth and tenderness

◆ Use of projection as a primary defense mechanism

■ Criteria for medical diagnosis (see the diagnostic criteria for paranoid personality disorder, page 152.)

■ Treatment

◆ Neuroleptic therapy

◆ Symptom management

Diagnostic criteria for personality disorders

This chart presents the *DSM-IV-TR* diagnostic criteria for the personality disorders discussed in this chapter. The criteria refer to behaviors or traits characteristic of the person's recent (past year) and long-term (generally since adolescence or early adulthood) functioning. These behaviors or traits cause subjective distress or significant impairment in social or occupational functioning. Behaviors or traits limited to episodes of illness are not considered when diagnosing a personality disorder.

Paranoid personality disorder

A. The person exhibits a pervasive distrust and suspiciousness of others, beginning by early adulthood and present in various contexts, to interpret the motives of others as malevolent, deliberately demeaning, or threatening as indicated by four or more of the following:
  1. Suspects, without sufficient basis, exploitation, or harm by others
  2. Questions, without justification, the loyalty or trustworthiness of friends or associates
  3. Is reluctant to confide in others because of unwarranted fear that the information will be used against him or her
  4. Reads hidden demeaning or threatening meanings into benign remarks or events (such as suspecting that a neighbor has put out the trash early to cause annoyance)
  5. Bears grudges or is unforgiving of insults or slights
  6. Perceives attacks on his character or reputation that are not apparent to others and is quick to react with anger or to counterattack
  7. Questions, without justification, fidelity of spouse or sexual partner

B. The disturbance does not occur exclusively during the course of schizophrenia, a mood disorder with psychotic features, or another psychotic disorder and is not due to direct physiological effects of a general medication condition.

Schizoid personality disorder

A. The person exhibits a pervasive pattern of detachment from social relationships and a restricted range of emotional experience and expression, beginning by early adulthood and present in various contexts, as indicated by four or more of the following:
  1. Neither desires nor enjoys close relationships, including being part of a family
  2. Almost always chooses solitary activities
  3. Has little, if any, desire to have sexual experiences with another person
  4. Takes pleasure in few, if any, activities
  5. Has no close friends or confidants (or only one) other than first-degree relatives
  6. Is indifferent to the praise and criticism of others
  7. Displays emotional coldness, detachment, or flattened affect

B. The disturbance does not occur exclusively during the course of schizophrenia, a mood disorder with psychotic features, or another psychotic disorder and is not due to the direct physiological effects of a general medical condition.

Schizotypal personality disorder

A. A pervasive pattern of social and interpersonal deficits marked by acute discomfort with, and reduced capacity for, close relationships as well as by cognitive or perceptual distortions and eccentricities of behavior, beginning by early adulthood and present in various contexts, as indicated by five or more of the following:
  1. Ideas of reference (excluding delusions of reference)
  2. Odd beliefs or magical thinking that influences behavior and is inconsistent with subcultural norms (such as superstition, belief in clairvoyance, telepathy or "sixth sense"; in children and adolescents, bizarre fantasies or preoccupations)
  3. Unusual perceptual experiences, such as bodily illusions (for example, believing that a body part is grotesque and belongs to a monster).
  4. Odd thinking and speech (such as speech that is circumstantial, metaphorical, overelaborate, stereotypical or vague)

Diagnostic criteria for personality disorders *(continued)*

    5. Suspiciousness or paranoid ideation
    6. Inappropriate or constricted affect (is silly or aloof; rarely reciprocates gestures or facial expressions, such as smiles or nods)
    7. Odd or eccentric behavior or appearance (is unkempt, displays unusual mannerisms, talks to self)
    8. Lacks close friends or confidants other than first-degree relatives
    9. Excessive social anxiety that does not diminish with familiarity and tends to be associated with paranoid fears rather than negative judgments about self
B. The disturbance does not occur exclusively during the course of schizophrenia, a mood disorder with psychotic features, another psychotic disorder or a pervasive developmental disorder

Antisocial personality disorder

A. There is a pervasive pattern of disregard for and violation of the rights of others occurring since age 15, as indicated by three or more of the following:
    1. Failure to conform to social norms with respect to lawful behaviors as indicated by repeatedly performing acts that are grounds for arrest
    2. Deceitfulness as indicated by repeatedly lying, using aliases, or conning others for personal profit or pleasure
    3. Impulsivity or failure to plan ahead
    4. Irritability and aggressiveness as indicated by repeated physical fights or assaults
    5. Reckless disregard for safety of self or others
    6. Consistent irresponsibility as indicated by repeated failure to sustain consistent work behavior or honor financial obligations
    7. Lack of remorse as indicated by being indifferent to or rationalizing having hurt, mistreated, or stolen from another
B. The individual is at least 18 years old
C. There is evidence of a conduct disorder with onset before age 15.
D. The occurrence of antisocial behavior is not exclusive to the course of a schizophrenic or manic episode.

Borderline personality disorder

The person exhibits a pervasive pattern of instability of interpersonal relationships, self-image and affects, and marked impulsivity, beginning by early adulthood and present in various contexts, as indicated by five or more of the following:
    1. Frantic efforts to avoid real or imagined abandonment (do not include suicidal or self-mutilating behavior covered in criterion 5)
    2. A pattern of unstable and intense interpersonal relationships characterized by alternating between extremes of idealization and devaluation
    3. Identity disturbance: markedly and persistently unstable self-image or sense of self
    4. Impulsivity in at least two areas that are potentially self-damaging (such as spending, sex, substance use, shoplifting, reckless driving, or binge eating; do not include suicidal or self-mutilating behavior covered in criterion 5)
    5. Recurrent suicidal threats, gestures, or behavior or self-mutilating behavior
    6. Affective instability due to a marked reactivity of mood (that is, intense episodic euphoria, irritability, or anxiety lasting a few hours and only rarely more than a few days), marked shifts from baseline mood to depression, irritability, or anxiety, usually lasting a few hours and only rarely more than a few days
    7. Chronic feelings of emptiness
    8. Inappropriate, intense anger or difficulty controlling anger (such as frequent displays of temper, constant anger, or recurrent physical fights)
    9. Transient, stress-related paranoid ideation or severe dissociative symptoms

Histrionic personality disorder

The person exhibits a pervasive pattern of excessive emotionality and attention-seeking, beginning by early adulthood and present in various contexts, as indicated by five or more of the following:

(continued)

Diagnostic criteria for personality disorders *(continued)*

1. Is uncomfortable in situations in which he or she is not the center of attention
2. Is inappropriately sexually seductive in appearance or behavior; exhibits provocative behavior in interaction with others
3. Displays rapidly shifting and shallow expression of emotions
4. Consistently uses physical appearance to draw attention to self
5. Has a style of speech that is excessively impressionistic and lacking in detail
6. Shows self-dramatization, theatricality, and exaggerated expression of emotion
7. Is easily influenced by others or circumstances
8. Considers relationships to be more intimate than they actually are

Narcissistic personality disorder

The person exhibits a pervasive pattern of grandiosity (in fantasy or behavior), lack of empathy, and need for admiration beginning by early adulthood and present in various contexts, as indicated by five or more of the following:

1. Has a grandiose sense of self-importance (for example, exaggerates achievements and talents; expects to be noticed as "special" without appropriate achievement)
2. Is preoccupied with fantasies of unlimited success, power, brilliance, beauty, or ideal love
3. Believes that he or she is "special" and unique and can only be understood by, or should associate with, other special or high status people (or institutions)
4. Requires excessive admiration
5. Has a sense of entitlement: that is, unreasonable expectations of especially favorable treatment or compliance with his or her expectations
6. Is interpersonally exploitative: that is, takes advantage of others to achieve his or her own ends
7. Lacks empathy; is unwilling to recognize or identify with the feelings and needs of others
8. Is often envious of others or believes that others are envious of him or her
9. Shows arrogant, haughty behaviors or attitudes

Avoidant personality disorder

The person exhibits a pervasive pattern of social inhibitions, feelings of inadequacy and hypersensitivity to negative evaluation, beginning by early adulthood and present in various contexts, as indicated by four or more of the following:

1. Avoids occupational activities that involve significant interpersonal contact because of fear of criticism, disapproval or rejection
2. Is unwilling to get involved with people unless certain of being liked
3. Shows restraint within intimate relationships because of the fear of being shamed or ridiculed
4. Is preoccupied with being criticized or rejected in social situations
5. Is inhibited in new interpersonal situations because of feelings of inadequacy
6. Views self as socially inept, personally unappealing, or inferior to others
7. Is unusually reluctant to take personal risks or to engage in any new activities because they may prove embarrassing

Dependent personality disorder

A pervasive and excessive need to be taken care of that leads to submissive and clinging behavior and fears of separation, beginning by early adulthood and present in various contexts, as indicated by five or more of the following:

1. Has difficulty making everyday decisions without an excessive amount of advice and reassurance from others
2. Needs others to assume responsibility for most major areas of his or her life
3. Has difficulty expressing disagreement with others because of fear of loss of support or approval.
   Note: Don't include realistic fears of retribution
4. Has difficulty initiating projects or doing things on his or her own (because of lack of self-confidence in judgment or abilities rather than a lack of motivation or energy)

Diagnostic criteria for personality disorders *(continued)*

5. Goes to excessive lengths to obtain nurturance and support from others, to the point of volunteering to do things that are unpleasant

6. Feels uncomfortable or helpless when alone because of exaggerated fears of being unable to care for himself

7. Urgently seeks another relationship as a source of care and support when a close relationship ends

8. Is unrealistically preoccupied with fears of being left to take care of himself

Obsessive-compulsive personality disorder

A pervasive pattern of preoccupation with orderliness, perfectionism, and mental and interpersonal control, at the expense of flexibility, openness, and efficiency, beginning by early adulthood and present in various contexts, as indicated by four or more of the following:

1. Is preoccupied with details, rules, lists, order, organization, or schedules to the extent that the major point of the activity is lost

2. Shows perfectionism that interferes with task completion (that is, is unable to complete a project because his or her own overly strict standards are not met)

3. Is excessively devoted to work and productivity to the exclusion of leisure activities and friendships (not accounted for by obvious economic necessity)

4. Is overconscientious, scrupulous, and inflexible about matters of morality, ethics, or values (not accounted for by culture or religious identification)

5. Is unable to discard worn-out or worthless objects even when they have no sentimental value

6. Is reluctant to delegate tasks or work with others unless they submit to exactly his or her way of doing things

7. Adopts a miserly spending style toward both self and others; money is viewed as something to be hoarded for future catastrophes

8. Shows rigidity and stubbornness

Adapted from *Diagnostic and Statistical Manual of Mental Disorders,* 4th ed., text revision, Washington, D.C.: American Psychiatric Association, 2000, with permission of the publisher.

◆ *Note:* Therapies that involve confrontation of feelings and alliances with others *aren't* effective
■ Selected nursing diagnoses
  ◆ Delayed growth and development related to unmet childhood needs
  ◆ Impaired parenting related to lack of knowledge about the parenting role
  ◆ Risk for other-directed violence related to antisocial character
  ◆ Fear related to being harmed by others
■ General nursing interventions
  ◆ Maintain an unambiguous environment
  ◆ Clarify the meanings and contexts of conversations, situations, and events
  ◆ Develop and nurture trust in the nurse-patient relationship

❖ **Schizoid personality disorder**
  ■ Characteristics
    ◆ Steadfast determination to remain distant and aloof

◆ Preference for solitary activities to those that require interaction with others
◆ Inability to form relationships, impoverished social skills, lack of desire to develop social contacts
◆ Emotionally restricted affect; rare (if any) expression of feelings
◆ Use of intellectualization as a primary defense mechanism
■ Criteria for medical diagnosis (see the diagnostic criteria for schizoid personality disorder, page 152)
■ Treatment: outpatient therapies designed to increase interpersonal comfort
■ Selected nursing diagnoses
◆ Deficient diversional activity related to unsustained social contact
◆ Social isolation related to aloof, withdrawn behavior
■ General nursing interventions
◆ Provide safety in the nurse-patient interaction
◆ Allow the physical and emotional space needed by the patient
◆ Foster the development of basic social skills (providing for the patient's daily needs should supercede diversional activity)

❖ **Schizotypal personality disorder**
■ Characteristics
◆ Eccentric behavior
◆ Expression of unusual ideas
◆ Magical thinking (belief that the person possesses special powers)
◆ Inability to form and maintain age-appropriate relationships
◆ Anxiety in social situations
◆ Dysphoria
■ Criteria for medical diagnosis (see the diagnostic criteria for schizotypal personality disorders, pages 152 and 153)
■ Treatment
◆ Neuroleptic therapy
◆ Social skills development
◆ Guidance in the management of daily affairs
◆ *Note:* Intensive psychotherapy generally isn't effective
■ Selected nursing diagnoses
◆ Ineffective role performance related to eccentric behavior
◆ Disturbed thought processes related to odd ideas
◆ Impaired social interaction related to anxiety
◆ Disturbed personal identity related to self-centered feelings
■ General nursing interventions
◆ Institute safety precautions
◆ Assist the patient in developing rudimentary social skills
◆ Help the patient with personal grooming and hygiene

❖ **Antisocial personality disorder**
  ■ Characteristics
    ◆ Consistent antisocial behavior (more common in males)
    ◆ Sustained history of irresponsibility and impulsiveness
    ◆ Lack of remorse for one's destructive actions
    ◆ Manipulation and exploitation of others
    ◆ Extreme self-centeredness
    ◆ Belief that one's actions are justified
    ◆ Anxiety and depression
    ◆ Anger that results in hostile outbursts
    ◆ Use of rationalization and acting out as primary defense mechanisms
  ■ Criteria for medical diagnosis (see the diagnostic criteria for antisocial personality disorder, page 153)
  ■ Treatment
    ◆ Group psychotherapy
    ◆ Confrontation of inappropriate behaviors
    ◆ Milieu conducive to generating feedback from peers
  ■ Selected nursing diagnoses
    ◆ Noncompliance (with treatment) related to the patient's denial of problems
    ◆ Risk for other-directed violence related to a disregard for the feelings of others
    ◆ Sexual dysfunction related to harmful relationships
    ◆ Impaired social interaction related to a disregard for the feelings or property of others
  ■ General nursing interventions
    ◆ Provide a stable environment
    ◆ Apply behavioral limits judiciously
    ◆ Assist the patient in taking responsibility for the consequences of actions
    ◆ Encourage the patient to verbalize hostile feelings
    ◆ Set consistent limits and provide a structured environment

❖ **Borderline personality disorder**
  ■ Characteristics
    ◆ Impulsiveness
    ◆ Outbursts of intense anger and rage
    ◆ Emotional lability
    ◆ Unstable identity
    ◆ Inability to be alone
    ◆ Self-mutilation
    ◆ Harmful, unstable, intense relationships
    ◆ Bouts of depression
    ◆ Anxiety
    ◆ Use of splitting, idealization, devaluation, and projective identification as primary defense mechanisms

- Criteria for medical diagnosis (see the diagnostic criteria for border-line personality disorder, page 153)
- Treatment
  - ◆ Group psychotherapy
  - ◆ Individual psychotherapy
  - ◆ Structured living under supervision
  - ◆ Neuroleptic therapy
- Selected nursing diagnoses
  - ◆ Ineffective coping related to unmet dependency needs
  - ◆ Chronic low self-esteem related to feelings of worthlessness
  - ◆ Disturbed personal identity related to identity uncertainty
  - ◆ Risk for self-directed violence related to parental or emotional deprivation
- General nursing interventions
  - ◆ Provide a structured, supportive, and consistent environment
  - ◆ Counter the patient's attempts to cause dissension among staff members
    - ▸ Adhere strictly to the treatment plan
    - ▸ Refuse to engage in third-party conversations
  - ◆ Encourage the patient to keep a journal to help him identify feelings

❖ Histrionic personality disorder
- Characteristics
  - ◆ Melodramatic, colorful, highly energetic personality
  - ◆ Development of shallow relationships
  - ◆ Tendency to make many demands on others for reassurance
  - ◆ Somatic complaints, marked by exaggeration of symptoms
  - ◆ Seductive, self-centered nature
  - ◆ Inability to establish genuinely intimate relationships
  - ◆ Bursts of exaggerated emotion in any situation
  - ◆ Use of somatization and dissociation as primary defense mechanisms
- Criteria for medical diagnosis (see the diagnostic criteria for histrionic personality disorder, pages 153 and 154)
- Treatment: outpatient supportive therapy
- Selected nursing diagnoses
  - ◆ Chronic low self-esteem related to unsatisfactory personal relationships
  - ◆ Impaired social interaction related to seductive behavior
  - ◆ Risk for other-directed violence related to poor impulse control
- General nursing interventions
  - ◆ Allay the patient's anxiety about meeting needs for love and affection
  - ◆ Teach the patient ways to delay needs for gratification
  - ◆ Assist the patient in assuming a mature adult role
  - ◆ Assist the patient in identifying feelings and in learning how to express them in a socially acceptable manner

❖ Narcissistic personality disorder
- ■ Characteristics
  - ◆ Inflated sense of self-importance
  - ◆ Feelings of entitlement to recognition
  - ◆ Craving and search for constant attention
  - ◆ Feelings of worthlessness if not lavishly praised and admired by others
  - ◆ Development of shallow interpersonal relationships based primarily on how others can meet the patient's needs for esteem
  - ◆ Lack of empathy
  - ◆ Depression
  - ◆ Rage
  - ◆ Shame and humiliation
  - ◆ Use of idealization as a primary defense mechanism
- ■ Criteria for medical diagnosis (see the diagnostic criteria for narcissistic personality disorder, page 154)
- ■ Treatment: individual or group therapy
- ■ Selected nursing diagnoses
  - ◆ Chronic low self-esteem related to feelings of worthlessness
  - ◆ Ineffective role performance related to demands for attention
  - ◆ Defensive coping related to grandiosity
- ■ General nursing interventions
  - ◆ Enhance the patient's self-esteem and sense of self-worth
  - ◆ Assist the patient in identifying feelings and in learning how to express them in a socially acceptable manner
  - ◆ Maintain a stable environment for the patient, and apply limits consistently
    - ❗ These interventions tend to enhance the person's sense of safety
    - ❗ They also can help reduce manipulative behaviors

❖ Avoidant personality disorder
- ■ Characteristics
  - ◆ Avoidance of any situation that could result in criticism
  - ◆ Hypersensitivity to rejection
  - ◆ Ineptitude and discomfort in social settings (social phobias may be evident), despite craving the interpersonal contacts the patient so fearfully shuns
  - ◆ Anxiety and depression
  - ◆ Anger
  - ◆ Use of avoidance as a primary defense mechanism
- ■ Criteria for medical diagnosis (see the diagnostic criteria for avoidant personality disorder, page 154)
- ■ Treatment
  - ◆ Assertiveness training
  - ◆ Social skills training
  - ◆ Relaxation exercises

- Selected nursing diagnoses
  - ◆ Social isolation related to shunning interpersonal contact
  - ◆ Anxiety related to the possibility of making social mistakes
  - ◆ Powerlessness related to helpless lifestyle
  - ◆ Chronic low self-esteem related to feelings of being unable to deal with life's events
- General nursing interventions
  - ◆ Enhance the patient's ability to confront social situations
  - ◆ Role-play events; then discuss what the patient thought would happen

❖ Dependent personality disorder
- Characteristics
  - ◆ Unassertiveness and passivity
  - ◆ Abdication of decision making to others
  - ◆ Belief that one won't be liked or will be abandoned if one offends another
  - ◆ Inability to take risks or to initiate anything without prior approval from others
  - ◆ Depression and anxiety
  - ◆ Use of self-devaluation as a defense mechanism
- Criteria for medical diagnosis (see the diagnostic criteria for dependent personality disorder, pages 154 and 155)
- Treatment
  - ◆ Assertiveness training
  - ◆ Relaxation exercises
- Selected nursing diagnoses
  - ◆ Impaired adjustment related to dependence on others
  - ◆ Decisional conflict (delayed decision making) related to lack of experience in making choices without help
  - ◆ Ineffective role performance related to fear of initiating actions
- General nursing interventions
  - ◆ Enhance the patient's ability to speak up and assume age-appropriate responsibilities
  - ◆ Give assignments that involve the patient in risk-taking behaviors

❖ Obsessive-compulsive personality disorder
- Characteristics
  - ◆ Preoccupation with order and rules
  - ◆ Perfectionism
  - ◆ Tendency to prescribe how others must do things
  - ◆ Inefficiency caused by constant worry over doing things correctly
  - ◆ Either anger or emotional constriction
  - ◆ Use of reaction formation, undoing, and displacement as primary defense mechanisms

■ Criteria for medical diagnosis (see the diagnostic criteria for obsessive-compulsive personality disorder, page 155)
■ Treatment
◆ Behavioral therapies
◆ Cognitive therapies
◆ Leisure activities
■ Selected nursing diagnoses
◆ Disturbed sleep pattern related to preoccupation with obsessive-compulsive behaviors
◆ Anxiety related to the need for perfection
◆ Ineffective health maintenance related to difficulty in completing activities of daily living
■ General nursing interventions
◆ Assist the patient in becoming more flexible and in generating alternative solutions to life situations
◆ Confront invalid assumptions so the patient can reassess a situation and develop a new perspective

Clinical situation

Kay, age 29, is admitted to your psychiatric unit for treatment and evaluation after an episode of self-mutilation. She inflicted the injury after her boyfriend of 1 week cancelled a date with her because he had to work late. Kay now has been on the unit for about 48 hours. During this time, she has had several angry outbursts about the doctors and nurses not being able to meet with her on demand. She vacillates between saying she wants to turn her life around and saying that she's a horrible person who should be allowed to die. Kay's diagnosis on admission is borderline personality disorder.

As Kay's primary nurse, you've contracted to spend two 30-minute blocks of time with her on an individual basis each day. However, Kay says she needs more time with you, and she manages to get you to spend up to 4 hours per shift with her by telling you that you're the only one she can trust, the only one who "really cares" about her.

Kay spends much of her time on the phone, complaining to friends about how badly she's being treated in the hospital. She also tries several times to contact her new boyfriend, and when her attempts prove unsuccessful, she uses profane language and throws a chair. When not on the phone, Kay hangs around the nurses' station, demanding to be seen, or sits in the day room with a male patient. Staff members have observed them holding hands, rubbing each other's back, and engaging in prolonged kissing. Kay is now demanding off-unit privileges because remaining on the unit is "boring as hell."

Assessment (nursing behaviors and rationales)

1. Assess Kay's potential for further self-mutilation and for suicide. *Ensuring the patient's safety is the nurse's top priority when caring for a patient with* *borderline personality disorder. Self-mutilation is a primary characteristic of this disorder, and suicide attempts are commonplace. Knowing the patient's state of mind about self-destruction provides data for planning appropriate care.*

2. Assess Kay's ability to control her impulses. *The patient's potential for acting-out behavior places her and others at risk for injury.*

3. Assess Kay's level of ego functioning. *This assessment provides information about the patient's strengths and weaknesses.*

4. Assess the effect that Kay is having on staff and other patients. *Power struggles are inevitable when caring for a patient with borderline personality disorder. Unless staff members remain clear on what needs to be addressed—and by whom, how, and when—the patient may succeed in causing dissension among the staff, which would be detrimental to all parties.*

Nursing diagnoses

- Risk for self-directed or other-directed violence related to poor impulse control
- Ineffective coping related to immature ego structure
- Noncompliance (with the treatment plan) related to power struggles between the patient and authority figures
- Impaired social interaction related to underlying fear of abandonment

Planning and goals

- Kay won't harm herself or others while hospitalized.
- She'll practice age-appropriate coping skills.
- She'll follow a written contract for compliance with treatment protocols.

Implementation (nursing behaviors and rationales)

1. Teach Kay problem-solving skills she can use to interrupt acting-out behaviors when feeling abandoned, lonely, afraid, or angry. *This helps the patient learn that her responses to situations are stimulated by underlying negative feelings that are related to external events. Such insight will probably empower the patient to remain in control.*

2. Provide Kay with a consistent environment by strictly adhering to the agreed-upon treatment plan and by using written contracts that you mutually review each day. *Such consistency creates a "holding" environment in which the patient can feel safe. Written contracts greatly reduce ambiguities and game playing. Daily review of the contracts promotes a consistent treatment approach, permits each party to clarify any misunderstandings, and allows for timely updating as needed.*

3. Hold daily staff conferences to address all problems that result from Kay's maladaptive behaviors. *Daily sessions severely curtail the patient's ability to cause dissension among staff members and provide the staff with a vehicle for airing concerns relating to the patient's care.*

4. Use rational authority when enforcing limits that are defined by unit policy or written contract. *Consistent, dispassionate limit-setting greatly enhances the patient's feelings of security, eventually eliminates power struggles,* *and ultimately increases the patient's ability to predict future events based on consistent past experiences. Furthermore, rational authority helps staff members avoid personalizing their actions or feeling responsible for the patient's behaviors or their consequences.*

5. Develop specific schedules for contacts between Kay and staff members. *Like other patients with borderline personality disorder, the patient in this clinical situation fears abandonment. She acts out and behaves inappropriately to compel others to be in her proximity. If she knows when to expect contact with staff, she may better tolerate the times when she must be alone.*

6. Specify the rules that Kay must follow when relating to other patients and the consequences she must face if she ignores the rules. *Staff members have an obligation to protect other patients from this patient's seductive ploys. Because of the nature of her illness, she's a master at exploiting others to meet her needs. They in turn are at risk for emotional or physical harm.*

Evaluation

- Kay doesn't harm herself or others while hospitalized.
- She learns to delay gratification by identifying her needs and by selecting rational, age-appropriate ways to meet these needs.
- She practices relaxation techniques when she becomes aware of feeling anxious.
- She participates in a support group for people with borderline personality disorder.
- She sets realistic daily goals.

Review questions

1. On admission to a surgical unit for treatment of a self-inflicted stab wound, the patient states, "Next time I'll do a better job. I don't want to be responsible for anyone's mistakes." The nurse's first response should be:

○ **A.** "I don't understand. What mistakes are you responsible for?"

○ **B.** "We are here to make sure nothing happens to you."

○ **C.** "Don't you realize how lucky you are that you survived this?"

○ **D.** "What exactly do you plan to do?"

Correct answer: D   The nurse must first assess the patient's potential for further self-mutilation and for suicide. After ensuring the patient's safety, the nurse can ask questions such as the one expressed in option A. The statement in option B offers the patient false reassurance. The question in option C shames the patient and minimizes her pain.

2. A 42-year-old computer analyst has difficulty with interpersonal relationships. His employer refers him to the local community mental health center. During his interview, the patient appears detached and claims he has no interest in the people at work. "They're all screwed up anyway," he says. He's single and comments further that he doesn't have the time or desire for a relationship. These behaviors indicate which of the following personality disorders?

○ **A.** Major depressive disorder

○ **B.** Obsessive-compulsive personality disorder

○ **C.** Conversion disorder

○ **D.** Schizoid personality disorder

Correct answer: D Patients suffering from schizoid personality disorder are cold and aloof and have no desire to be in a relationship. Major depressive disorder and conversion disorder aren't personality disorders. Symptoms of obsessive-compulsive personality disorder include rigid adherence to rules and perfectionism. Although they tend to be very anxious, people with obsessive-compulsive personality disorder can form meaningful relationships.

3. The nurse is assessing a patient with a personality disorder. Which of the following assessment information is most important to elicit?

○ **A.** a family history of sexual abuse

○ **B.** socioeconomic background

○ **C.** ability to form close relationships

○ **D.** history of substance abuse

Correct answer: D Patients with personality disorders frequently have a history of substance abuse because they have difficulty controlling impulses and managing their feelings. A nurse needs to know about the patient's history of substance abuse in order to assess his safety and potential for going through withdrawal. After determining the patient's history of substance abuse, the nurse can assess his ability to form close relationships and his family history of sexual abuse. Socioeconomic background isn't vital to treatment.

4. The police bring a tarot card reader into treatment after she becomes belligerent with a customer who questioned her "reading." The patient is oriented to reality but discloses that she can read the nurse's mind. The patient's behavior is typical of which of the following personality disorders?

○ **A.** Narcissistic personality disorder

○ **B.** Schizotypal personality disorder

○ **C.** Paranoid personality disorder

○ **D.** Antisocial personality disorder

Correct answer: B Common symptoms of schizotypal personality disorder include magical thinking and eccentric behavior. Paranoid patients tend to have suspicious rather than magical thoughts. Typical symptoms of an antisocial personality include disregard for the rights of others and criminal activity; magical thinking isn't usually evident. The patient's symptoms don't meet the criteria for narcissistic personality disorder.

5. The most helpful therapeutic intervention for an antisocial patient is:

   ○ **A.** to allow special privileges to assure the patient that the nurse is empathetic.

   ○ **B.** to offer direct feedback from peers in a milieu setting.

   ○ **C.** to prescribe hypnosis and guided meditation.

   ○ **D.** to prescribe antianxiety medication.

Correct answer: B Antisocial patients respond better to feedback from peers than to a person in authority. Allowing special privileges is contraindicated for antisocial patients because they already believe they're above the law. Hypnosis and guided meditation wouldn't be helpful for an antisocial patient because such therapies don't provide the patient the opportunity to interact with others. Pharmacological intervention is contraindicated (unless the patient is extremely agitated or aggressive) because antianxiety agents can be addictive. Hypnosis and guided meditation don't allow the patient interaction with others.

Schizophrenia

❖ **Overview**
  ■ Schizophrenia is the most commonly diagnosed thought disorder
  ■ It's characterized by severe, prolonged disturbances of affect; withdrawal from reality; regressive behavior; poor communications; and impaired interpersonal relationships (see *Diagnostic criteria for schizophrenia*, page 167)
  ■ Onset begins with a notable impairment in some areas of daily functioning, such as work, social relationships, and self-care
  ■ The person's premorbid personality is usually described as suspicious, introverted, withdrawn, eccentric, and impulsive
  ■ The person reports feeling "strange," is confused about the origin of the impairment, and develops a sense of being separate and different from others
  ■ Life expectancy among those with schizophrenia is shortened because of an increased likelihood of suicide
  ■ The disorder usually begins during adolescence or early adulthood but can develop in middle or late adulthood

❖ **Theoretical perspectives**
  ■ Biological theories
    ◆ Genetic theory
      ▶ Although the specific genetic defect hasn't been identified, researchers believe chromosome 6 is a factor in schizophrenia (chromosomes 4, 8, 15 and 22 may also contribute)
      ▶ If one parent has schizophrenia, the child has a 15% risk of developing it; if both parents have the disease the risk goes up to 35%
      ▶ For identical twins, the risk of both members of the pair developing schizophrenia is 35% to 70% greater than the general population
    ◆ Neurobiological theory
      ▶ Multiple studies (including computed tomography and magnetic resonance imaging) show anatomical, functional, and neurochemical abnormalities in brains of people with schizophrenia
      ▶ Dopamine causes overactive neuronal activity; drugs that decrease dopamine activity decrease psychotic symptoms
      ▶ An imbalance between dopamine and serotonin appears in the brain

Diagnostic criteria for schizophrenia

This chart presents the *DSM-IV-TR* diagnostic criteria for schizophrenia.

A. *Characteristic symptoms:* The person exhibits two or more of the following, each present for a significant portion of time during a 1-month period (or less if successfully treated):
1. Delusions
2. Hallucinations
3. Disorganized speech (such as frequent derailment or incoherence)
4. Grossly disorganized or catatonic behavior
5. Negative symptoms (affective flattening, alogia, or avolition)

Note: Only one criterion A symptom is required if delusions are bizarre or if hallucinations consist of either one voice keeping up a running commentary on the person's behavior or thoughts or two or more voices conversing with each other.

B. *Social/occupational dysfunction:* For a significant portion of time since onset of the disturbance, one or more major areas of functioning (such as work, interpersonal relations, or self-care) are markedly below the level achieved before the onset (or, when the onset is in childhood or adolescence, failure to achieve expected level of interpersonal, academic, or occupational achievement).

C. *Duration:* Continuous signs of the disturbance persist for 6 months or more. This 6-month period must include 1 month or more (or less if successfully treated) of symptoms that meet criterion A (characteristic symptoms) and may include periods of prodromal or residual symptoms. During these prodromal or residual periods, signs of the disturbance may be manifested by only negative symptoms or by two or more symptoms listed in criterion A that are present in an attenuated form (such as odd beliefs or unusual perceptual experiences).

D. *Schizoaffective and mood disorder exclusion:* Schizoaffective disorder and mood disorder with psychotic features have been ruled out because either (1) no major depressive, manic, or mixed episodes have occurred concurrently with characteristic symptoms or (2) if mood episodes have occurred during characteristic symptoms, their total duration has been brief relative to the duration of the active and residual periods.

E. *Substance/general medical condition exclusion:* The disturbance is not due to the direct physiologic effects of a substance (such as a drug of abuse or a medication) or a general medical condition.

F. *Relationship to a pervasive developmental disorder:* If the patient has a history of autistic disorder or another pervasive developmental disorder, the additional diagnosis of schizophrenia is made only if prominent delusions or hallucinations are also present for 1 month or more (or less if successfully treated).

Classification of a longitudinal course (can be applied only after 1 year or more has elapsed since initial onset of characteristic symptoms):

Episodic with Interepisode Residual Symptoms (episodes are defined by the reemergence of prominent psychotic symptoms); *also specify if:* **With Prominent Negative Symptoms**
Episodic with No Interepisode Residual Symptoms
Continuous (prominent psychotic symptoms are present throughout observation); *also specify if:* **With Prominent Negative Symptoms**
Single Episode in Full Remission
Other or Unspecified Pattern

Adapted from *Diagnostic and Statistical Manual of Mental Disorders*, 4th ed., text revision, Washington, D.C.: American Psychiatric Association, 2000, with permission of the publisher.

◆ Neurodevelopmental theory
▶ Multiple structural, functional, and chemical brain deviations are present before symptoms appear
▶ Cause of the deviations could be genetic programming, environmental injury or both
◆ Viral theories
▶ Prenatal exposure to the influenza virus may be a factor in the development of schizophrenia

▶ How the virus affects a developing fetus to cause symptoms is unknown
■ Biosocioenvironmental theory
◆ The interaction between the individual and the environment influences the development of the disorder
◆ The occurrence of schizophrenia is related to the environment and to one's inner strength and vulnerability to stress

❖ **Signs and symptoms**
■ Language and communications disturbances
◆ A person with schizophrenia can't maintain a consistent, logical train of thought
◆ Reasoning usually follows the person's own unfathomable private rules
◆ The person shows poverty of speech and may begin to form neologisms in severe stages of the disorder
■ Thought disturbances
◆ Delusions, particularly those about the person's thoughts being read by others, are characteristic
◆ Ideas of reference and persecution delusions are intense
■ Perceptual disturbances
◆ Auditory hallucinations are the most common type
◆ Voices communicate directly with the person, criticizing the person's thoughts and behavior
■ Affect disturbances
◆ The demonstrable emotion is labile or flat and commonly is inappropriate
◆ The person typically complains of losing "normal feelings"
■ Motor behavior disturbances
◆ The person may be in a state of constant, wildly bizarre, and aggressive activity that can lead to profound exhaustion
◆ Conversely, the motor disturbance can produce a marked decrease in activity, leading to a virtual cessation of spontaneous movement (catatonia)
■ Self-identity disturbances
◆ The person loses a sense of self-identity
◆ The person believes that mysterious forces are changing the person's core being; a sense of nothingness develops

❖ **Subtypes of schizophrenia**
■ Paranoid type
◆ Primary characteristics include persecutory delusions and hallucinations
◆ Communications break down because of the person's extreme suspicion, which leads to reduced levels of functioning and withdrawn behavior

- Catatonic type
  - ◆ The primary characteristic is either increased motor excitement or stuporous, rigid, posturing behavior
  - ◆ The extreme withdrawal helps the person control fear and anxiety
- Disorganized type
  - ◆ Primary characteristics include incoherent speech, unsystematized delusions, and inappropriate, flat affect
  - ◆ The disturbance produces marked functional impairment with a poor outlook for remission
- Undifferentiated type
  - ◆ Primary characteristics include grossly disorganized, incoherent behavior; hallucinations; and prominent delusions
  - ◆ The person's functioning level is severely impaired
- Residual type
  - ◆ The primary characteristic is a lack of schizophrenic symptoms, although the person has had a schizophrenic episode
  - ◆ Functioning level is moderate, but the person seldom can keep a job

❖ Treatment
- Psychosocial therapy
  - ◆ This form of therapy initially focuses on the patient's physical safety
  - ◆ Once the patient's safety has been established, health care personnel form a therapeutic alliance with the patient to understand the patient's behavior and to support the patient in abandoning maladaptive behaviors for more acceptable ones
  - ◆ Therapists then design a treatment plan to raise the patient's functioning level and to educate the family on how to respond to the patient's behavior
  - ◆ A team approach — one that involves a psychiatrist or psychologist, a nurse, and a social worker — is used to carry out the treatment plan
- Drug therapy
  - ◆ Phenothiazine and neuroleptic agents have been remarkably effective in restoring the patient's functioning level so that the patient can return to society
  - ◆ Drug treatment may consist of low-potency or high-potency drugs, depending on the treatment strategies adopted to relieve psychotic symptoms
  - ◆ Adjunctive drugs, such as anticholinergic agents, propranolol, and diphenhydramine, may be used to control adverse effects
- Combination therapy
  - ◆ Although drug treatment can help normalize a patient's behavior, it has marginal effect on improving the patient's social skills or overall quality of life
  - ◆ Long-term treatment requires building a stable psychological foundation and helping the patient accept responsibility for self-care, the development of social relationships, and vocational satisfaction

❖ Selected nursing diagnoses
- Disturbed thought processes related to inability to trust, an underdeveloped ego, and biochemical imbalances
- Ineffective coping related to low self-esteem
- Social isolation related to lack of trust and delusional thinking
- Dressing/grooming self-care deficit related to regression to an earlier developmental level
- Disturbed sensory perception (visual) related to hallucinations
- Impaired verbal communication related to withdrawn behavior
- Risk for other-directed violence related to suspiciousness
- Noncompliance (with the treatment plan) related to suspiciousness and lack of insight

❖ General nursing interventions
- Safety
  - ◆ Remove any unsafe objects from the patient's environment
  - ◆ Reassure the patient that the environment is safe by explaining procedures used to provide protection
  - ◆ Monitor the patient for increased psychomotor activity, intensity of affect, and verbalization or carrying out of delusional thinking
- Environment
  - ◆ Keep the patient oriented to reality
  - ◆ Minimize environmental stimuli
  - ◆ Reassure other patients that their behavior did not provoke the patient's threats
  - ◆ Communicate in clear, direct, and concise statements
- Self-esteem
  - ◆ Assist the patient with grooming, if needed
  - ◆ Allow the patient to make decisions when appropriate
  - ◆ Acknowledge the patient's abilities and skills, and use them to reinforce teaching
- Social activities
  - ◆ Assist the patient in identifying lifestyle patterns that can be used to build better social relationships
  - ◆ Help the patient evaluate the effectiveness of communication skills and social interactions
  - ◆ Give positive reinforcement when the patient voluntarily interacts with others
  - ◆ Encourage the patient to participate in group activities
- Ego development
  - ◆ Validate the patient's perceptions that are accurate, and correct misperceptions
  - ◆ Spend time with the patient even when the patient can't respond coherently
  - ◆ Convey acceptance of the patient while attempting to correct unacceptable behavior

◆ Give praise and encouragement when the patient chooses socially acceptable methods of managing anger and aggression
■ Homeostasis
◆ Monitor the patient's vital signs
◆ Provide periods for adequate sleep
◆ Provide a nutritious diet
◆ Control hyperactive psychomotor activity

Clinical situation

John Ellis, age 36, is admitted to your psychiatric unit for the third time with a diagnosis of schizophrenia. The day before, he had been arrested for intimately touching a woman he didn't know, without her consent. Then, while in jail awaiting arraignment, he burned himself with matches he had hidden. The injury required treatment at the local hospital's emergency department, where he reportedly hit his father, who had come to see him.

Now, on arrival at the psychiatric facility, John is in handcuffs, yelling repeatedly. He appears restless, agitated, demanding, suspicious, and paranoid, and he exhibits looseness of association. John admits to auditory hallucinations and seems out of contact with reality. For the past year, according to his medical records, he has been taking chlorpromazine (Thorazine) 100 mg b.i.d., trifluoperazine (Stelazine) 20 mg b.i.d., and benztropine (Cogentin) 1 mg in the morning.

Assessment (nursing behaviors and rationales)

1. Assess John's potential for violence against others or self. *If the patient exhibits suicidal tendencies or overt hostile and aggressive behaviors, the nurse and other staff members will need to take precautions to protect the patient and others from harm.*

2. Assess John's personal hygiene, sleep pattern, and motor activity level. *This assessment provides data that the nurse can use to determine the amount of nursing assistance the patient requires.*

3. Assess John's coping pattern, social support, financial status, educational level, and patterns of interactions with others. *This assessment provides information about perceived and actual coping ability, developmental level, and problem-solving ability. It also helps determine the availability of family and friends to assist in the patient's recovery.*

4. Assess the type of hallucinations and delusions that John is experiencing. *Information obtained from this assessment reveals the extent of the patient's disorganized thinking.*

5. Assess for adverse effects of antipsychotics. *Adverse effects include akathisia, dystonia, parkinsonism, neuroleptic malignant syndrome, tardive dyskinesia, anticholinergic effects, weight gain and sexual difficulties.*

6. Conduct a thorough physical examination. *A physical examination provides data about possible organic causes for behavior.*

Nursing diagnoses

- Disturbed thought processes related to impaired judgment
- Disturbed sensory perception (auditory) related to hallucinations
- Social isolation related to distrust of others
- Risk for self-directed violence related to lack of trust and delusional thinking
- Dressing/grooming self-care deficit related to withdrawn behavior and inattention to personal grooming

Planning and goals

- John will remain oriented to reality by controlling his behavior.
- He'll maintain a satisfactory balance of nutritious diet, adequate sleep, and proper exercise.
- He won't harm others or himself.
- He'll participate in the therapeutic environment.

Implementation (nursing behaviors and rationales)

1. Focus the patient on reality. Don't reinforce delusional thinking, but acknowledge its presence. *Acknowledging delusional thinking and searching for what might have triggered it are the first steps toward defusing it.*

2. Provide for uninterrupted sleep as much as possible. *With adequate sleep, the patient will experience less physical and psychological stress and exhibit fewer bizarre behaviors.*

3. Establish a pattern of therapeutic communication. *Effective communication can facilitate the development of the therapeutic nurse-patient relationship and help the patient in working through the problem-solving process.*

4. Monitor vital signs and provide for John's physical needs. *Systematic monitoring alerts the nurse to a change in the patient's functional status and the need for prompt intervention.*

5. Don't argue with John about his delusions or hallucinations. *Altered perceptions frighten the patient and indicate loss of control. Because of lack of insight, this patient views his delusions and hallucinations as reality. Arguing only leads to defensiveness.*

6. Establish a daily routine for John. *The patient's ability to adapt is severely impaired. A well-maintained routine is less threatening to him.*

7. Monitor the frequency of hallucinations and the intensity of delusions. *Command hallucinations or delusions may precede bizarre, destructive, or suicidal behavior.*

8. Teach John basic social skills such as conversation. *The patient may never have learned how to carry on a social conversation, such as discussing the weather or a sporting event. Developing basic social skills can help build the patient's self-confidence, enhance self-esteem, and reduce anxiety, all of which contribute to social acceptance.*

9. Direct John toward activities that will decrease the likelihood of his acting on hallucinatory or delusional misinterpretations. *Redirecting the pa-*

tient's energies to more acceptable activities helps reduce the likelihood of inappropriate behavior.

10. Provide opportunities for John to accept responsibility and make decisions. *The patient must gain a sense of independence before he can be discharged. Accepting responsibility for behavior and participating in decision making enhance the patient's self-confidence and promote his sense of independence.*

11. Teach John and family members about John's condition. Review the importance of taking medications as prescribed, and discuss their adverse effects. *To ensure proper care at home and to promote compliance with treatment, the patient and his family must have accurate information about his illness, treatment, and effects of medications.*

Evaluation

- John follows an adequate diet and maintains a proper balance of sleep and exercise.
- He demonstrates increased self-esteem.
- He becomes independent in self-care.
- He engages in community social activities.
- He accurately repeats the instructions for taking his medication and can recite their adverse effects.

Review questions

1. Schizophrenia is characterized by which of the following?

○ **A.** Short but severe disturbances of affect

○ **B.** Withdrawal from reality

○ **C.** Aggressive and assertive behavior

○ **D.** Few interpersonal relationships

Correct answer: B Withdrawal from reality is the principal characteristic of schizophrenia. In addition, the patient exhibits severe, prolonged disturbances of affect, regressive behavior, and impaired interpersonal relationships.

2. An individual who displays stuporous, rigid posturing behavior and extreme withdrawal is exhibiting which of the following types of schizophrenia?

○ **A.** Catatonic type

○ **B.** Paranoid type

○ **C.** Disorganized type

○ **D.** Residual type

Correct answer: A   Extreme withdrawal and rigid posturing behavior are characteristics of catatonic type schizophrenia. Paranoid type schizophrenia is characterized by persecutory delusions and hallucinations. Characteristics of disorganized type schizophrenia include incoherent speech, unsystematized delusion, and inappropriate, flat affect. Individuals with residual type schizophrenia tend to lack schizophrenic symptoms, although the person has experienced a schizophrenic episode.

3. Which of the following nursing actions would be most appropriate for a delusional patient?

○ **A.** Focus the patient on reality.

○ **B.** Refute the delusion.

○ **C.** Explain that the patient's feelings are common.

○ **D.** Explore the patient's feelings.

Correct answer: A   It's important to keep a delusional patient focused on reality. Don't reinforce delusional thinking, but acknowledge its presence. Acknowledging delusional thinking and searching for what might have triggered it are the first steps in defusing such thinking. Explaining that the patient's feelings are common or exploring the patient's feelings don't directly address the delusion.

4. A patient with hallucinations and intense delusions should be monitored closely for which of the following?

○ **A.** Depression

○ **B.** Regression

○ **C.** Suicidal behavior

○ **D.** Injury to others

Correct answer: C   Command hallucinations or delusions (for example, those that tell the patient to hurt himself) should alert the nurse to the patient's potential for self-destructive behavior. This behavior is typically self-directed and doesn't pose a risk of injury to others. Although depression and regression are also concerns for a patient experiencing hallucinations or delusions, monitoring the patient's potential for self-destructive behavior is the highest priority.

Somatoform disorders

❖ **Overview**
- Somatoform disorders are a group of psychological conditions characterized by complaints of physical symptoms or illness for which no organic or physiologic cause exists
- The patient typically has a lengthy history of diagnostic workups with negative physical findings, leading the health care professional to suspect a psychological cause for the physical symptoms
- The patient doesn't have conscious control of the symptoms, which feel real to the patient
- The psychological origin of these disorders is thought to be repressed anxiety
  - ◆ The primary gain is that the symptoms allow the patient to avoid the awareness of an internal conflict or need
  - ◆ The symptoms represent, and partially solve, an underlying conflict
- Symptom formation and apparent disability are reinforced by a secondary gain, in which the person avoids a particularly unpleasant action and elicits support from others
- Patients with somatoform disorders are commonly seen first by doctors for treatment of perceived medical symptoms
- The differentiating diagnostic factor is the absence of any physiologic origin for the symptoms

❖ **Theoretical perspectives**
- Psychoanalytic theory
  - ◆ Freud postulated that successful psychological development depended on satisfying specific physical functions, such as eating or toilet training
  - ◆ Physical symptoms in somatoform disorders signal intrapsychic conflict from failure to meet earlier developmental needs
- Genetic theory
  - ◆ Studies suggest an increased incidence of somatoform disorders in females who have first-degree relatives with the disorder
  - ◆ Researchers are still investigating the potential link between genetics and somatoform disorders

■ Family dynamics theory
  ◆ Family members are unable to openly express emotions and verbally resolve problems
  ◆ Illness within the family provides a stabilizing force; the family shifts its focus from internal conflicts to the illness.
  ◆ The illness provides positive reinforcement of the patient's physical symptoms
■ Holistic theory
  ◆ Mental and physiologic processes are directly linked
  ◆ Any illness is physical and psychological, each affecting the other
■ Stress theory
  ◆ Stress, even unconscious stress, can cause psychophysiologic disorders
  ◆ Selye syndrome, generalized adaptation syndrome, proposes three levels of response to stress
    ▶ *Alarm reaction:* the body is put into a "fight or flight" stance
    ▶ *Stage of resistance:* the body reduces its optimum level of function
    ▶ *Stage of exhaustion:* the body's adaptive ability fails, and death becomes imminent

❖ **Body dysmorphic disorder**
  ■ Characteristics
    ◆ Preoccupation with an imaginary defect in one's physical appearance, even though the person appears normal to others
    ◆ Complaints of facial flaws (or flaws in other parts of the body)
    ◆ Slight physical abnormality, but the person's preoccupation with it is out of proportion to the magnitude of the abnormality
    ◆ Primary incidence in young people beginning in adolescence
    ◆ Tendency to seek unnecessary surgery to correct the imaginary defect or minor flaw
    ◆ Possible impairment of social skills and work performance resulting from the patient's desire to hide the perceived flaw
  ■ Criteria for medical diagnosis (see the diagnostic criteria for body dysmorphic disorder, page 177)
  ■ Treatment
    ◆ Cognitive or other forms of psychotherapy
    ◆ Psychotropic medication to relieve associated depression and anxiety
  ■ Selected nursing diagnoses
    ◆ Disturbed body image related to perceived disfigurement
    ◆ Ineffective coping related to inadequate coping skills and low self-esteem
    ◆ Anxiety related to perceived physical flaw
    ◆ Risk for injury related to unnecessary surgery
  ■ General nursing interventions
    ◆ Listen to the patient's complaints empathetically

Diagnostic criteria for somatoform disorders

This chart presents the *DSM-IV-TR* diagnostic criteria for the somatoform disorders discussed in this chapter.

Body dysmorphic disorder

A. The person has a preoccupation with an imagined defect in appearance. If a slight physical anomaly is present, the person's concern is markedly excessive
B. The preoccupation causes clinically significant distress or impairment in social, occupational, or other important areas of functioning
C. The preoccupation is not better accounted for by another mental disorder (for example, dissatisfaction with body shape and size in anorexia nervosa)

Conversion disorder

A. The person has one or more symptoms or deficits affecting voluntary motor or sensory function that suggest a neurologic or other general medical condition
B. Psychological factors are judged to be associated with the symptom or deficit because the initiation or exacerbation of the symptom or deficit is preceded by conflicts or other stressors
C. The symptom or deficit is not intentionally produced or feigned (as in factitious disorder of malingering)
D. The symptom or deficit cannot, after appropriate investigation, be fully explained by a general medical condition or the direct effects of a substance or be described as a culturally sanctioned behavior or experience
E. The symptom or deficit causes clinically significant distress or impairment in social, occupational, or other important areas of functioning or warrants medical evaluation
F. The symptom or deficit is not limited to pain or sexual dysfunction, does not occur exclusively during the course of somatization disorder, and is not better accounted for by another mental disorder

Hypochondriasis

A. Preoccupation with fears of having, or the idea that one has, a serious disease based on the person's misinterpretation of bodily symptoms
B. The preoccupation persists despite appropriate medical evaluation and reassurance
C. The belief in criterion A is not of delusional intensity (as in delusional disorder, somatic type) and is not restricted to a circumscribed concern about appearance (as in body dysmorphic disorder)
D. The preoccupation causes clinically significant distress or impairment in social, occupational, or other important areas of functioning
E. The duration of the disturbance is at least 6 months
F. The preoccupation is not better accounted for by generalized anxiety disorder, obsessive-compulsive disorder, panic disorder, a major depressive episode, separation anxiety, or another somatoform disorder
Specify if:
With Poor Insight: If, for most of the time during the current episode, the person does not recognize that the concern about having a serious illness is excessive or unreasonable

Pain disorder

A. Pain in one or more anatomical sites is the predominant focus of the clinical presentation and is of sufficient severity to warrant clinical attention
B. The pain causes clinically significant distress or impairment in social, occupational, or other important areas of functioning
C. Psychological factors are judged to have an important role in the onset, severity, exacerbation, or maintenance of the pain
D. The symptom or deficit is not intentionally produced or feigned (as in factitious disorder or malingering)
E. The pain is not better accounted for by a mood, anxiety, or psychotic disorder and does not meet criteria for dyspareunia

(continued)

Diagnostic criteria for somatoform disorders (continued)

Somatization disorder

A. The person has a history of many physical complaints beginning before age 30 that occur over several years and result in treatment being sought or significant impairment in social, occupational, or other important areas of functioning

B. Each of the following criteria must have been met, with individual symptoms occurring at any time during the course of the disturbance:

   1. *Four pain symptoms:* a history of pain related to at least four different sites or functions (for example, head, abdomen, back, joints, extremities, chest, rectum; during menstruation, sexual intercourse, or urination)

   2. *Two gastrointestinal symptoms:* a history of at least two gastrointestinal symptoms other than pain (such as nausea, bloating, vomiting other than during pregnancy, diarrhea, or intolerance of several different foods)

   3. *One sexual symptom:* a history of at least one sexual or reproductive symptom other than pain (sexual indifference, erectile or ejaculatory dysfunction, irregular menses, excessive menstrual bleeding, vomiting throughout pregnancy)

   4. *One pseudoneurologic symptom:* a history of at least one symptom or deficit suggesting a neurologic condition not limited to pain (conversion symptoms such as impaired coordination or balance, paralysis or localized weakness, difficulty swallowing or lump in throat, aphonia, urine retention, hallucinations, loss of touch or pain sensation, double vision, blindness, deafness, seizures; dissociative symptoms such as amnesia; or loss of consciousness other than fainting)

C. The condition is characterized by either of the following:

   1. After appropriate investigation, each of the symptoms in criterion B cannot be fully explained by a known general medical condition or the direct effects of a substance (such as a drug of abuse or a medication)

   2. When the patient has a related general medical condition, the physical complaints or resulting social or occupational impairments are in excess of what would be expected from the history, physical examination, or laboratory findings

D. The symptoms are not intentionally produced or feigned (as in factitious disorder or malingering)

Adapted from *Diagnostic and Statistical Manual of Mental Disorders,* 4th ed., text revision, Washington, D.C.: American Psychiatric Association, 2000, with permission of the publisher.

◆ Support the patient's attempts to acknowledge that the existence or extent of the defect may be exaggerated

◆ Accompany the patient to activities that are too uncomfortable for the patient to attend alone

◆ Administer prescribed medications, and teach the patient about their adverse effects

❖ **Conversion disorder**
■ Characteristics
  ◆ Alteration or loss of functioning of a body part that isn't related to any physical abnormalities
  ◆ Symptoms not under the patient's conscious control
    ▶ May be either disturbing to the patient or not acknowledged (la belle indifference)
    ▶ Classically mimic neurologic problems, such as paralysis, blindness, aphonia, and other sensory disturbances
    ▶ May involve GI or other systems
    ▶ Appear to express a conflict or an unmet need; primary and secondary gains are in operation

▶ Can be a single symptom of a presenting illness that may migrate or vary in subsequent episodes

▶ Can be multiple symptoms that severely constrict the patient's ability to function, resulting in actual physical impairment from disuse of the body part

■ Criteria for medical diagnosis (see the diagnostic criteria for conversion disorder, page 177)

■ Treatment

◆ Thorough physical workup for each new presenting symptom

◆ Psychotherapy to enable the patient to acknowledge and resolve unconscious conflict

◆ Physical rehabilitation for muscle atrophy, if indicated

◆ Medication to relieve associated anxiety and depression

■ Selected nursing diagnoses

◆ Disturbed sensory perception (kinesthetic) related to repressed anxiety

◆ Bathing/hygiene self-care deficit related to impaired ability to perform or complete activities of daily living independently.

◆ Risk for disuse syndrome related to loss of function of body part

◆ Disabled family coping related to disturbed family relations

◆ Ineffective coping related to feelings of inadequacy

◆ Ineffective role performance related to physical conversion symptom

■ General nursing interventions

◆ Allow the patient to express feelings; listen empathetically and nonjudgmentally

◆ Monitor and report any new conversion symptoms

◆ Encourage independence with self-care and assist with basic physiologic needs (such as eating, hygiene, safety)

◆ Provide a safe environment for the patient's particular impairment

◆ Monitor for suicide potential

◆ Support the family as they attempt to provide encouragement without providing secondary gain

❖ Hypochondriasis

■ Characteristics

◆ Morbid preoccupation with a fear or belief that one has a serious disease based on a personal interpretation of physical health

◆ No physical evidence of serious disease

◆ Unwavering conviction of illness; the patient is neither delusional nor preoccupied with bodily functions

◆ Anxiety, depression, and compulsive behavior

◆ Avoidance of responsibility

◆ Desire for attention

◆ Manipulation of others

■ Criteria for medical diagnosis (see the diagnostic criteria for hypochondriasis, page 177)

■ Treatment
 ◆ Thorough physical examination and workup for each new conversion episode or complaint
 ◆ Psychotherapy, with the frequency of sessions related to the patient's level of anxiety
 ◆ Medication to reduce associated anxiety and depression
 ◆ Relaxation techniques
■ Selected nursing diagnoses
 ◆ Fear (of having a serious illness) related to past experiences with life-threatening illness.
 ◆ Ineffective coping related to denial of emotional problems
 ◆ Anxiety related to ineffective coping ability
 ◆ Ineffective health maintenance related to preoccupation with body functions
 ◆ Risk for disuse syndrome from loss of function of a body part
 ◆ Deficient knowledge (illness) related to denial process
■ General nursing interventions
 ◆ Recognize the physical complaint as being real to the patient
 ◆ Identify gains, such as gaining attention and avoiding responsibility, that the patient's physical symptoms may support
 ◆ Allow the patient to express concerns about physical symptoms; assume a nonjudgmental attitude
 ◆ Offer the patient health teaching about the illness, when appropriate
 ◆ Teach and demonstrate relaxation techniques and other coping skills
 ◆ Monitor and report any new conversion signs or symptoms
 ◆ Monitor for suicide potential

❖ **Somatization disorder**
 ■ Characteristics
 ◆ Many physical complaints or an ongoing conviction of serious illness beginning before age 30 and occurring over many years
 ◆ Dramatic but often vague communication of somatic complaints
 ◆ Lack of organic or physiologic cause for symptoms
 ◆ Possible appearance of other psychiatric diagnoses, such as anxiety and depression
 ■ Criteria for medical diagnosis (see the diagnostic criteria for somatization disorder, page 178)
 ■ Treatment
 ◆ Thorough physical workup for each symptom
 ◆ Genuine understanding by the health care professional that although no physical cause may be evident, the patient's distress and impairment are real and not consciously caused or controlled
 ◆ Psychotherapy to assist the patient in dealing with unconscious conflicts and anxiety
 ◆ Antidepressants and antianxiety medications, if prescribed

■ Selected nursing diagnoses
  ◆ Noncompliance (with treatment) related to secondary gain from being sick
  ◆ Ineffective coping related to use of physical illness as coping mechanism
  ◆ Deficient knowledge (of diagnosis and treatment) related to inadequate understanding of the disorder
  ◆ Chronic low self-esteem related to unsatisfactory interpersonal relationships
■ General nursing interventions
  ◆ Monitor and report any new signs or symptoms
  ◆ Listen objectively to the patient, neither encouraging nor discouraging the expression of the patient's symptoms
  ◆ Discuss with the patient a possible connection between emotions and physical symptoms
  ◆ Protect the patient's right to treatment and respect
  ◆ Discuss the patient's expectations about being in the hospital
  ◆ Involve the patient in planning care, setting goals, and selecting interventions

❖ **Pain disorder**
  ■ Characteristics
    ◆ Preoccupation with pain without any diagnostic finding to account for the pain or its intensity
    ◆ Pain that doesn't follow anatomical nervous system distribution (although the pain does feel real to the person and isn't consciously feigned)
    ◆ Long history of physical complaints, consultations with numerous doctors, drug or alcohol abuse, and marked impairment of lifestyle
    ◆ Clear connection between a psychological stressor and onset of symptoms
    ◆ Possible secondary gain as a motivating factor in developing symptoms
  ■ Criteria for medical diagnosis (see the diagnostic criteria for pain disorder, page 177)
  ■ Treatment: Individual psychotherapy (most common approach in the absence of a definitive treatment for this condition)
  ■ Selected nursing diagnoses
    ◆ Chronic pain related to repressed anxiety and learned maladaptive coping skills
    ◆ Ineffective coping related to repressed anxiety and unmet dependency needs
    ◆ Social isolation related to preoccupation with self and pain
    ◆ Ineffective role performance related to continual search for medical attention

- General nursing interventions
  - ◆ Monitor laboratory results and assess any new signs or symptoms
  - ◆ Teach and reinforce relaxation techniques and alternative coping skills
  - ◆ Acknowledge that the patient is actually experiencing pain and distress while encouraging the patient to explore feelings
  - ◆ Reduce the opportunity for secondary gain by encouraging the patient to perform as much self-care as possible
  - ◆ Administer pain medication as ordered; provide comfort measures as appropriate

Clinical situation

Tom, age 17, is brought to the local emergency room after sustaining an injury while playing football at his homecoming game. He exhibits paralysis from his waist to his toes. A neurologist is consulted and tests reveal no organic etiology for the paralysis. Tom is diagnosed with conversion disorder and is admitted to the mental health unit.

Tom's interactions with others on the unit demonstrate that he has good social skills, and he makes friends very easily. He doesn't mention his paralysis and acts as if everything is just fine. His attitude is that of la belle indifference.

His family, friends, and girlfriend visit frequently. Information gathered from the family reveals that Tom was the all-star player on the football team. He was also nominated for king of the homecoming court.

Tom is referred to physical therapy so he can learn to use a wheelchair and implement an exercise regime to maintain his muscle tone. He attends group therapy and tells the group that he doesn't understand what happened to him — one minute he was perfectly fine and the next he was paralyzed. He says that he doesn't think he needs to be on a "psych" unit because he's not crazy.

Assessment (nursing behaviors and rationales)

1. Perform a nursing assessment. *A nursing assessment establishes baseline physical, psychosocial, and cultural data that can be used to develop an individualized treatment plan.*
2. Assess Tom's level of disability. *This information will be used to plan patient care.*
3. Assess Tom's perception of his situation. *Perception may help guide the interventions.*

Nursing diagnoses

- Disturbed sensory perception (kinesthetic) related to repressed anxiety
- Bathing/hygiene self-care deficit related to alteration in physical functioning (paralysis)
- Ineffective coping related to feelings of inadequacy

Planning and goals

- Tom will demonstrate recovery of altered physical function
- He'll be able to perform self-care activities independently
- He'll be able to verbalize a connection between stress and symptoms

Implementation (nursing behaviors and rationales)

1. Don't focus on the paralysis, and encourage independence with activities. Intervene when necessary. *Positive reinforcement will encourage maladaptive behaviors.*

2. Maintain a nonjudgmental attitude when assisting Tom. *The patient's symptoms are unconscious. A judgmental attitude will interfere with the therapeutic relationship.*

3. Encourage Tom to verbalize his anxiety and fears and assist him with implementing coping mechanisms in stressful situations. *Patients are usually unaware of the psychological implications of their illness.*

4. Encourage Tom to disclose and explore his feelings. *Discussing feelings in a trusting, therapeutic relationship may help fulfill unmet needs and confront unresolved issues.*

Evaluation

- Tom demonstrates recovery from physical disability.
- Tom is able to verbalize a connection between his loss of function and the stressful event.
- He's able to demonstrate more adaptive coping skills to deal with stress or conflict.
- He's able to identify resources outside the hospital setting when in need of assistance.

Review questions

1. A 25-year-old mother of two children visits the clinical nurse specialist for outpatient therapy. Although slender, the woman has a slight bulge in her lower abdomen, and she's seeking treatment "because of my huge stomach." She mentions how self-conscious she is of her stomach and says that she doesn't look right in any of her clothing. The woman is showing signs and symptoms of which disorder?

○ **A.** Somatization disorder

○ **B.** Body dysmorphic disorder

○ **C.** Conversion disorder

○ **D.** Hypochondriasis

Correct answer: B Individuals with body dysmorphic disorder grossly exaggerate a slight physical anomaly. Patients with somatization disorder tend to have many physical complaints or an ongoing conviction of serious illness, but they lack a physical cause for their symptoms. An alteration or loss of functioning of a body part that isn't related to physical abnormalities suggests conversion disorder. Characteristics of hypochondriasis include a fear or belief that one has a serious disease (although no physical evidence of disease exists), anxiety, depression, and compulsive behavior.

2. A 9-year-old boy is admitted to the mental health unit for conversion disorder. He exhibits total paralysis while standing in place like a statue. He typically takes 20 minutes to get to group therapy because he repeatedly becomes frozen in action. What's the nurse's best response when he displays this behavior?

○ **A.** "I'll call for someone to bring a wheelchair to escort you to the group."

○ **B.** "Going to group therapy is hard work. I'll wait for you until you're able to continue walking to the group."

○ **C.** "This is ridiculous. Everyone knows there's nothing wrong with you."

○ **D.** "I'll come back later when you're able to walk to the group."

Correct answer: B The patient needs to take the initiative to physically bring himself to therapy. By encouraging the patient to attend group therapy, the nurse helps motivate him to acknowledge and confront the unconscious conflict causing his physical symptoms. Staying with the patient until he's able to continue walking provides the patient with support and feelings of self-worth. Leaving the patient may be interpreted as abandonment. To put the patient in a wheelchair negates the patient's goal to get to therapy on his own. Telling the patient that nothing is wrong with him is not therapeutic.

3. A woman, age 36, has been diagnosed with hypochondriasis. Which of the following symptoms would the nurse expect her to display?

○ **A.** Grossly exaggerated perception of a slight physical anomaly

○ **B.** Loss of a bodily function

○ **C.** Attitude of la belle indifference

○ **D.** Unwavering conviction of illness

Correct answer: D Hypochondriacs typically believe they have a serious illness, despite lack of physical evidence of disease. Individuals with the disorder seek many medical opinions even though previous doctors have reported negative findings. Grossly exaggerated perception of a slight physical anomaly is more characteristic of body dysmorphic disorder. Loss of bodily function and attitude of la belle indifference are related to conversion disorder.

4. What's considered the first priority when treating conversion disorder, somatization disorder, and hypochondriasis?

○ **A.** Assisting the patient with basic needs

○ **B.** Confronting the patient's underlying conflict

○ **C.** Performing a thorough physical workup of the presenting symptom

○ **D.** Preventing secondary gain

Correct answer: C A thorough physical workup of the symptom or complaint is essential to rule out organic etiology. After a thorough physical workup is completed, the patient may be assisted in meeting basic needs if he is unable to do so himself. Once physical illness is ruled out, therapy may begin to help the patient identify the underlying conflict as well as prevent secondary gain.

5. A patient is being treated for pain disorder. He has a 10-year history of back pain without successful treatment. Which of the following nursing diagnoses is most appropriate for this patient?

○ **A.** Chronic pain related to repressed anxiety and maladaptive coping skills

○ **B.** Deficient knowledge (of diagnosis and treatment) related to inadequate understanding of the disorder

○ **C.** Self-care deficit (hygiene) related to inability to perform acts of daily living independently

○ **D.** Fear (of having a serious illness) related to past experiences of life-threatening illnesses

Correct answer: A Chronic pain is typically related to repressed feelings and inadequate coping skills. This is the primary underlying dynamic of pain disorder. There's no information available in this situation to substantiate a nursing diagnosis of knowledge deficit, self care deficit, or fear.

Psychiatric therapies

❖ **Overview**
- Health care professionals use various therapies to treat psychiatric disorders
- The patient may be involved in a single therapeutic modality or a combination of treatment approaches, such as individual, group, family, milieu, and electroconvulsive therapy (ECT)
- Psychiatric theoretical models discussed earlier in this book are utilized in each therapeutic approach; for example, individual psychotherapy can utilize crisis intervention theory, Peplau's concepts of anxiety, and behavioral theory; and group and family therapy can integrate the psychoanalytic model and communication theory
- The patient's needs and the therapist's skills determine the treatment modality used

❖ **Individual therapies**
- Gestalt therapy
  - ◆ First developed in the 1940s, gestalt therapy has personal self-growth as its primary goal
  - ◆ Focusing on self-awareness, the therapist facilitates the patient's ability to engage in self-discovery
  - ◆ The therapist points out discrepancies in the patient's behavior and thoughts, without interpreting the behavior or thoughts
  - ◆ The patient is encouraged to set personal goals in life and to make independent choices
  - ◆ Gestalt therapy is based on several assumptions
    - ▶ Humans naturally strive to grow and satisfy basic needs
    - ▶ Self-awareness is central to meeting those needs
    - ▶ Reality is whatever is happening now
    - ▶ Focusing on the past or looking to the future prevents one from being totally in the present
    - ▶ To be fully empowered, a person must take total responsibility for making choices in life
  - ◆ Gestalt therapy relies on two therapeutic techniques
    - ▶ *Empty chair dialogue:* Using an empty chair, the patient is asked to imagine that a significant other or a past experience is in the chair;

the patient then engages in a "dialogue with the chair," with the therapist listening, observing, and calling attention to the patient's nonverbal communications

▶ *Dream discussion:* The patient recalls a dream and then acts out every character and event in the dream; dreams are considered a spontaneous psychic production containing an existential message

■ Psychoanalysis

◆ Psychoanalysis is a daily process of examining the working of the mind, using free association and dream analysis

◆ The patient is instructed to refrain from all activity during the 50-minute session so that all energy is focused on discovering mental content through verbalization

◆ The analyst seeks verbal patterns that provide insight into the patient's intrapsychic conflicts

◆ Dreams, fantasies, wishes, fears, and feelings are discussed during the analysis

◆ The analyst interprets the meaning of the dreams, fantasies, wishes, fears, and feelings, conscious and unconscious, to help the patient see the connection between unconscious wishes and conscious behavior

◆ The analyst-patient interaction produces *transference* (the strong emotional response that the patient develops toward the therapist) and *countertransference* (the analyst's emotional response to the patient)

◆ Success of the analysis depends on successful interpretation of the patient's mental content

◆ The patient gains insight on how to rework unresolved problems and adopt more adaptive solutions

◆ Psychoanalysis is a long-term therapy that requires a major time and financial commitment from the patient

■ Transactional analysis

◆ A theoretical communications model as well as a therapy, transactional analysis examines the communications (transactions) occurring between people, attempting to discover how people relate to one another

◆ It's based on several assumptions

▶ People make current life decisions based on past assumptions that are invalid

▶ Present-day life is restricted because of earlier invalid decisions

▶ Developing an awareness of how present-day life has been influenced by past assumptions enables the patient to change behavior

◆ The therapist works with the patient to analyze the three levels of ego communication

▶ *Complementary transaction level:* a healthy form of communication occurring between the ego states of adult to adult or child to child

▶ *Crossed transaction level:* a nonproductive form of communication between the ego states of adult to child or child to adult

❱ *Ulterior transaction level:* a destructive form of communication during which one person attempts to feel superior to another
◆ During transactional analysis, the patient is taught how to identify the ego state from which he operates and how to interrupt an automatic tendency to engage in nonproductive or destructive transactions
◆ The goal of therapy is to promote the use of the complementary transaction level to build maximum patient growth

■ Rational emotive therapy
◆ This type of therapy attempts to correct maladaptive behavior by changing established patterns of thinking that arise from underlying irrational thoughts, such as "I must be loved by everyone," "A woman without a man is nothing," or "If things go wrong, it's a catastrophe"
◆ Irrational learned responses are culture-specific
◆ The therapist's role is to help the patient gain three insights
❱ Irrational beliefs cause current misery; people disturb themselves
❱ An irrational belief is reinforced each time it's used
❱ The best way to change an irrational belief is to do something different; talking about it is ineffective
◆ During the sessions, the therapist aggressively points out and challenges the patient's irrational thoughts
◆ The goal of rational emotive therapy is to achieve happiness in life by thinking rationally and by accepting one's strengths and weaknesses

■ Reality therapy
◆ Reality therapy focuses on helping the patient meet needs by taking effective control over choices in life
◆ It assumes that human behavior is driven by needs; consequently, when one's needs aren't satisfied, one experiences pain
◆ People who meet their needs are successful and happy most of the time; those who don't meet their needs experience failure and pain
◆ The patient is constantly confronted during therapy with questions that reinforce self-responsibility, such as "What do you want?" or "What do you think is best?"
◆ The therapist refrains from giving advice

■ Individual psychotherapy
◆ This type of therapy establishes a relationship between the therapist and the patient in an attempt to understand the patient's intrapsychic conflicts
◆ Treatment is aimed at maintaining or modifying adaptive patterns and changing parts of the personality structure to build more effective adaptive behaviors
◆ Individual psychotherapy uses two major techniques

▶ *Supportive psychotherapy* strengthens the patient's inner defenses to help reduce anxiety; especially effective with patients who have a weak ego structure

▶ *Analytic psychotherapy* uses the interpretation of dreams, free association, and transference distortions to uncover intrapsychic conflicts

◆ Psychotherapy is most effective when the patient's problem is stress-related and the patient has the capacity to engage, work through, and disengage the treatment process

■ Behavior modification

◆ The therapist uses a five-step approach to change the patient's maladaptive behaviors

▶ Using direct observation, the therapist assesses the patient for symptoms of behavioral dysfunction (for instance, stuttering, crying, or inappropriate verbalizations, such as expressions of suicide ideation)

▶ The therapist then discusses treatment goals with the patient, focusing on specific behaviors that need changing

▶ Next, the therapist assesses the conditions that either promote or minimize these behaviors (behavioral analysis)

▶ The therapist then alters the patient's environment to effect changes in the patient's behavior

▶ Finally, the therapist observes, documents, and analyzes any behavioral changes that occur, and either continues the treatment as planned or develops alternative treatments

◆ Behavior modification is based on testing one hypothesis, which may lead to another, which also must be tested

◆ Therapists can use several techniques to modify behavior

▶ *Systematic desensitization*

● The patient learns relaxation techniques and new behaviors that can assist in reducing anxiety

● The patient learns to tolerate increasing amounts of anxiety

▶ *Graded exposure*

● The patient gradually makes contact with the source of the anxiety

● The patient learns that the anxiety-producing object is really harmless

● Eventually, the object no longer arouses intolerable amounts of anxiety

▶ *Social skills training*

● The therapist rewards the patient only for desirable social behaviors

● The therapist uses group role-playing and modeling to teach social skills

● Between sessions, the patient must complete homework assignments to practice and reinforce desirable behaviors

▶ *Response prevention*
  ● The therapist asks the patient to hesitate briefly before responding, in a characteristic way, to a noxious stimulus
  ● The therapist then models alternative responses to the stimulus
  ● The patient is rewarded for delaying the characteristic response
  ● Over time, the patient learns to tolerate noxious stimuli without immediately resorting to characteristic maladaptive responses
▶ *Token economy*
  ● The therapist provides the patient with a list of acceptable behaviors to a stimulus, along with the consequences of exhibiting undesirable behaviors
  ● For each acceptable behavior exhibited, the therapist awards the patient a token, which the patient can exchange for desired goods
  ● Over time, the patient learns acceptable behaviors

❖ **Group therapies**
  ■ Group psychotherapy
    ◆ This type of therapy is based on the premise that group influence is a powerful vehicle for structuring and reinforcing behavior
    ◆ It can be a treatment for many disorders that involve erroneous thinking or distortions of mental perceptions
    ◆ Group psychotherapy emphasizes the examination of interpersonal relationships; as in individual therapy, the patient's ego strength determines which therapeutic technique — supportive or analytic — is used
    ◆ Central concepts of group psychotherapy include the following:
      ▶ *Content* refers to what's said in the group
      ▶ *Process* refers to what's done in the group
      ▶ *Cohesiveness* refers to the sense of belonging that keeps all members in the group
      ▶ Other important concepts include *transference* and *countertransference* (see "Individual therapies," page 186) and *resistance* (forestalling the therapeutic process)
    ◆ Yalom developed 11 curative therapeutic factors of group therapy
      ▶ *Cohesion:* Group members support and accept the group as a unit
      ▶ *Catharsis:* The patient expresses his feelings in a nonthreatening environment
      ▶ *Universality:* The patient understands that some of his problems aren't unique; other patients may have similar problems and share common experiences
      ▶ *Altruism:* The patient is able to help others in the group, which supports his self-growth
      ▶ *Interpersonal learning:* Interpersonal skills learned within the group translate to the patient's relationships outside of the group
      ▶ *Identification*: The patient imitates the healthy behaviors of other group members in order to develop such behaviors in himself

▶ *Instillation of hope:* The patient develops a positive outlook while in group therapy

▶ *Recapitulation of primary family group:* The patient in group therapy is influenced by his history; when the patient works out problems with the other members of the group, he's also working through issues from his past

▶ *Insight:* The patient understands how he got to be how he is and why he does what he does

▶ *Imparting information:* By sharing and receiving feedback within the group, the patient achieves personal growth

▶ *Development of socialization techniques:* The patient is able to adhere to social norms

◆ Dynamics of a group include the following:

▶ *Rank* refers to the position of a member in the group

▶ *Status* refers to the prestige of a member in the group

▶ *Norms* are the group's rules of conduct or standards for appropriate behavior

▶ *Role* refers to the function or part that a member assumes within the group

◆ Every group should serve some therapeutic purpose; common purposes among groups in psychotherapy include the following:

▶ Personality reconstruction

▶ Remotivation and reeducation

▶ Support

▶ Problem solving

◆ Specialty groups are those consisting of patients with a commonality, such as age, gender, or educational background

◆ All groups must be led by a therapist knowledgeable about group dynamics and process

■ Family therapy

◆ Family therapy is directed toward liberating the patient from living in an environment in which there's acting out of family anxieties and conflicts

◆ A therapist meets with the family and attempts to focus on the patterns of family interaction, to reveal family secrets and myths, and to examine and make explicit their nonverbal communications

◆ Goals of family therapy are to minimize conflict, to build awareness of others among the members, and to help individual members deal with internal and external destructive processes

◆ Central concepts of family therapy include the following:

▶ *Triangles:* introduction of a third person into an uncomfortable interaction between two family members, to reduce the tension; a triangle can also be formed around an issue, an object, or a group

▶ *Multigenerational patterns:* process through which behavioral patterns are transmitted from one generation to another; a genogram is used to map out these patterns of interaction and behavior

▶ *Communication:* family interaction is considered in relation to how family members send, receive, and respond to verbal and nonverbal messages

▶ *Family system:* the whole is more than the sum of its parts; the system can be either functional or dysfunctional, based on its level of differentiation

▶ *Differentiation:* measurement of human functioning on a continuum, from a lower level of strong intensity of emotional fusion to an upper level of complete differentiation and emotional autonomy

  • A person at the lower level has emotions so fused with those of other family members that the person exhibits little emotional autonomy

  • A person at the upper level is emotionally and intellectually separated from other family members and is more adaptable to and independent of the emotions that surround the family

▶ *Family projection process:* projection of a family problem onto one or more children in the family (a process used by spouses to avoid marital confrontations)

▶ *Sibling position:* the place and role within the family that a child learns and assumes

■ Psychodrama

◆ This type of therapy uses structured and controlled dramatization of a patient's problems

◆ The goal is to dramatize emotional problems so they can be reexperienced and examined in a new way

◆ The therapy group provides immediate feedback to the actor (patient) so that new learning can occur

◆ Psychodrama can be cathartic in that the patient, after reliving past experiences and the emotions they generated, can rework the emotions in the present time to produce a more acceptable response

◆ Psychodrama consists of three phases

  ▶ *Warm-up*

    • The group decides which issue to explore
    • A protagonist (principal actor) is urged to come forward

  ▶ *Action*

    • The actors discuss the play to be enacted
    • The play begins
    • The actors spontaneously portray the roles assigned to them

  ▶ *Postaction group sharing*

    • The group members (actors) discuss personal experiences that the drama has reactivated
    • The members integrate their current feelings with those they once had toward the experiences
    • They search for new meaning in the awareness they have developed

◆ The techniques used in psychodrama are designed to enhance self-exploration and understanding

◆ Psychodrama can be effective in dealing with interpersonal conflicts such as marital discord

❖ Rehabilitation therapies

■ Occupational therapy

◆ Occupational therapy is the art and science of guiding a patient's participation in crafts and related activities to promote recovery from illness and maintain good health

◆ Such programs may involve an individual or a group and may be simple or complex; an occupational activities assessment determines the activity level selected for the patient

◆ Traditional occupational therapy activities include sewing, weaving, clay sculpturing, and the making of wood and leather artifacts; occupational therapists also participate in teaching daily living skills and other rehabilitation therapies, such as pet therapy and plant therapy

■ Art therapy

◆ Art therapy is the use of art to help a patient express feelings and inner conflicts

◆ In addition to being a form of treatment, it can be a diagnostic tool (for instance, the therapist may interpret the symbolism in a patient's drawings)

◆ Encouraging a patient to draw relieves anxiety and aggression in a socially acceptable way

■ Recreational therapy

◆ Recreational therapy is the use of controlled and planned physical activity to promote a patient's well-being and comfort

◆ It's based on the theory that a positive relationship between one's self and the environment contributes to good health

◆ The goals are to provide an outlet for energy release, to teach the patient how to play, to teach cooperation with others, and to help the patient develop leisure-time pursuits

◆ Recreational activities may be vigorous (such as dance, basketball, or tennis) or less strenuous (such as checkers or chess)

◆ The recreational therapist also identifies community resources that help integrate a discharged patient back into society

■ Play therapy

◆ Play therapy is the use of play as a means of communicating with children who have mental health problems

◆ It assumes that children younger than age 12 can express themselves better through the manipulation of objects (toys) than through words

◆ Observing a child at play provides clues about the child's developmental level, style of interaction, and areas of potential psychic conflict

◆ Children engage in five types of play
  ▶ *Exploratory:* The child experiments with different play techniques
  ▶ *Creative:* The child uses objects creatively
  ▶ *Diversional:* The child's activities have no purpose, indicating boredom
  ▶ *Mimetic:* The child attempts to master a skill by observing repetitive activity
  ▶ *Cathartic:* The play is hard, intense, and without pleasure; activities symbolize underlying stress

◆ Play development has three stages
  ▶ *Solitary (infant to toddler):* The child plays alone, unaware of others in the immediate environment
  ▶ *Parallel (toddler to school-age child):* The child plays near others but not with them
  ▶ *Cooperative (school-age child and older):* The child participates in organized play with others

◆ Play therapy has several benefits
  ▶ Promotes self-expression and creativity
  ▶ Discharges tension and aggression
  ▶ Enables the child to learn techniques for pleasure
  ▶ Fosters trust among those at play
  ▶ Permits expression of emotionally charged feelings

❖ **Other psychiatric therapies**
  ■ ECT
  ◆ An electric current passes through electrodes applied to the patient's temples to induce a generalized tonic-clonic seizure and unconsciousness
  ◆ It's used to treat patients with depression; bipolar I disorder, manic phase; and psychotic symptoms
  ◆ Nursing interventions for patients undergoing ECT include the following:
    ▶ Provide nothing by mouth after midnight to prevent vomiting during treatment
    ▶ Remove all prostheses, including dentures
    ▶ Dress the patient in loose-fitting clothing
    ▶ Teach the patient and family about the treatment and what to expect; explain the procedure and describe the short-term memory loss the patient can experience for several days after the procedure
    ▶ Obtain a signed informed consent
    ▶ Provide close observation immediately after the treatment
    ▶ Use the same nursing care procedures as for an unconscious patient

- Biofeedback
  - ◆ Biofeedback teaches the patient to bring body functions, such as blood pressure, heart rate, and skin temperature under conscious control
  - ◆ By controlling physical functions, the patient can relieve health problems, such as headaches, insomnia, chronic pain, or anxiety
  - ◆ Electronic equipment measures biological changes and signals the patient when such changes occur
  - ◆ There are four steps to biofeedback training
    - ▶ Awareness of the changes that occur before and during the designated health problem
    - ▶ Recognition of internal changes associated with specific symptoms
    - ▶ Learning to voluntarily alter the internal changes
    - ▶ Becoming motivated to learn biofeedback.
- Psychoeducation
  - ◆ Psychoeducation is the use of educational principles and techniques to rehabilitate and treat psychiatric patients
  - ◆ It's used to teach patients and their families about the patient's illness
  - ◆ It fosters collaboration and active participation in the treatment program
  - ◆ Patients who are exposed to psychoeducation learn information that helps them improve the quality of their lives; families learn how to accept and cope with a patient's illness, minimizing stress for all concerned
- Milieu therapy
  - ◆ Milieu therapy aims to treat a mental disorder by manipulating the patient's environment and focusing on the atmosphere of treatment
  - ◆ Its effectiveness depends on the attitudes of the health care team and their interaction with the patient
  - ◆ Through self-government, the patient assumes some responsibility for the management of the unit on which he lives
  - ◆ The unit is structured to provide human relationships that satisfy emotional needs, reduce psychological conflicts and deprivation, and strengthen impaired ego functions
  - ◆ Characteristics of a therapeutic milieu include the following:
    - ▶ The patient and staff share responsibility for care, including such issues as passes, discharges, and status changes
    - ▶ Role relationships are examined to determine which behaviors are appropriate
    - ▶ Staff members have ultimate authority for making decisions and establishing policies
    - ▶ Socialization and group interaction are emphasized in order to provide the best opportunity for living and learning

◆ The primary goal of milieu therapy is to provide an atmosphere in which the patient can learn to live a productive and successful life in society

◆ The nurse's role is a central component of milieu therapy because nurses are present on the unit 24 hours per day

Review questions

1. Which of the following principles would the nurse use to guide interventions that are based on Gestalt therapy?

○ **A.** People need to satisfy their basic needs.

○ **B.** Behavioral patterns are transmitted from generation to generation.

○ **C.** Care is designed to test hypotheses about health.

○ **D.** Families must practice relaxation techniques.

Correct answer: A Gestalt therapy is based on the principle that human beings will strive to grow and find ways to satisfy their basic needs. Family therapy is based on the principle that behavioral patterns are transmitted from generation to generation. Care is designed to encourage the patient to make independent decisions and set goals, not to test hypotheses. Relaxation techniques are used by the patient (not the family) in behavior modification therapy.

2. A psychiatric patient is depressed and is demanding of family members. Which of the following is an effective nursing intervention for directing the family?

○ **A.** Instruct the family to do everything for the patient.

○ **B.** Tell the family members not to intervene.

○ **C.** Teach the patient about self-care and self-awareness.

○ **D.** Explain to the family how to perform reality-testing with the patient.

Correct answer: C Teaching the patient self-care and self-awareness empowers the patient's family to create a healthy environment in which he can become functional and learn to handle the anxieties of daily living more effectively. Instructing the family to do everything for the patient isn't therapeutic. The family must be taught how to intervene with the patient. It isn't within the family's knowledge base to perform reality-testing; this is the therapist's responsibility.

3. What's the primary reason for using family therapy?

   ○ **A.** The identified patient isn't the only "sick" member of the family.

   ○ **B.** The family behaves as a system, each member influencing and responding to each other.

   ○ **C.** The marital relationship is the axis around which all other family relationships are formed.

   ○ **D.** The family needs to understand and learn to cope with the "sick" member's behavior.

   Correct answer: B   Family therapy allows the nurse to help the family see how each member contributes to the problem that needs resolution. Individuals in family therapy are not singled out as the "sick" member of the family. The family system is seen as a whole in which each member is a part. The family doesn't revolve around a particular relationship, such as the marital relationship.

4. At the end of a group therapy session, the nurse summarizes the discussion by saying, "From what I've been hearing, everyone is concerned about the recent absences of group members and the disruption of late-arriving members is causing frustration." Which of the following is the purpose of the nurse's statement?

   ○ **A.** To focus on the group content

   ○ **B.** To work on the group process

   ○ **C.** To clarify the group norms

   ○ **D.** To provide an example of how to share feelings

   Correct answer: C   The nurse focuses on the group's norms in order to establish the standards for appropriate group behavior. Group content refers to what's actually said during the group therapy session. The group process refers to what's done in the group. The nurse's statement doesn't refer to specific feelings, so it isn't an example of how to share feelings.

Psychopharmacology

❖ **Overview**

■ Before the early 1950s, the care of mentally ill people consisted primarily of removing them from families and loved ones and placing them indefinitely in extremely crowded institutions, where treatment may or may not have been provided

   ◆ Crude treatment modalities—such as insulin shock therapy; non-medicated electroconvulsive therapy; frontal lobe lobotomy; and the use of "cold packs," straight jackets, and padded cells—were the only "therapeutic interventions" available to treat symptoms of psychosis and depression

   ◆ The history of how these interventions were administered on such a vulnerable population contains documented evidence of inhumane attitudes and physical abuse, a legacy that today haunts not only the field of psychiatry and its practitioners but also those seeking treatment for mental distress

■ A milestone in the treatment of mental disorders occurred with the introduction of chlorpromazine (Thorazine) to therapeutic regimens

   ◆ The drug, discovered in France in the early 1950s, was initially used as a preoperative medication to lower anxiety

   ◆ Clinicians noted calmness, marked indifference to surroundings, and lowered body temperature in patients who received it

   ◆ Dr. Henri Laborit of the Boucicaut hospital in Paris suggested the application of chlorpromazine in psychiatry

   ◆ In 1955, clinicians in the United States began administering the drug to patients with psychotic and schizophrenic symptoms, particularly to those who exhibited violent behavior

   ◆ Clinicians observed significant improvement among such patients, as evidenced by a notable decline in violent and unruly behavior

■ Such behavioral improvements heightened the concerns of families and, eventually, politicians that institutionalization was preventing many humans from living to their fullest potential

■ The Joint Commission on Mental Health and Mental Illness prompted the establishment of the federal Community Mental Health Centers Act, which was passed in 1963

   ◆ Under that law, President Kennedy proposed a "bold new approach" to the treatment of mental disorders, one that emphasized returning hospitalized patients to active rehabilitation services in the community

◆ This proposal, which sparked what became known as the "Deinstitutionalization Movement," was made possible by the advent of medications for the treatment of mental disorders

■ Other advancements in science and technology have paved the way for continued improvements in treatment

◆ Greater understanding of the complexities of brain functioning and its relationship to psychiatric illness and modern therapy led scientists to recognize the significance of dopamine receptors and their effects on psychosis; this discovery challenged the traditional psychodynamic view of "poor nurturing" as being the sole cause of mental illness

◆ Sophisticated technology, such as positron emission tomography (PET), has allowed scientists to examine brain physiology and neurochemical actions in human beings

 ◗ Increased density of dopamine receptors in nontreated schizophrenics has been observed through the use of the PET scan

 ◗ These findings show a direct correlation between neurochemical actions in the brain and the role they play in psychiatric illness

■ Although they can provide symptom relief, psychotropic medications aren't a cure for mental illness; they should always be used as an adjunct to other psychotherapeutic interventions (see *Managing the adverse effects of psychotropic drugs,* pages 200 and 201)

❖ Antipsychotic drugs
 ■ Indications
  ◆ Acute and chronic psychosis associated with depression, schizophrenia, and post traumatic stress
  ◆ Bipolar I disorder, manic phase
  ◆ Paranoia
  ◆ Severe nausea and vomiting (antiemetic)
  ◆ Control of tics associated with Tourette's syndrome
 ■ Mechanism of action
  ◆ Block dopamine receptors in the central nervous system (basal ganglia, limbic system, hypothalamus, brain stem, and medulla), thereby reducing psychotic symptoms
  ◆ Block adrenergic and muscarinic receptors and exert an effect on other transmitters, such as gamma-aminobutyric acid, and peptides
 ■ Absorption, distribution, and elimination (see *Profile of antipsychotic drugs,* pages 202 and 203)
  ◆ Most antipsychotic medications are available in tablet, syrup, and injectable forms
   ◗ Liquid preparations are absorbed more rapidly than tablets
   ◗ Parenteral administration is absorbed rapidly, with the initial drug effect occurring within 15 minutes; peak plasma level occurs within 60 minutes

Managing the adverse effects of psychotropic drugs

Although psychotropic drugs can dramatically improve the health status of a patient with a psychiatric problem, their adverse effects can produce problems. These may range from minor discomforts, such as dry mouth, to more serious conditions, such as tardive dyskinesia and neuroleptic malignant syndrome. This chart presents common adverse effects of psychotropic drugs, along with appropriate nursing interventions.

Adverse effects	Nursing interventions
Drowsiness, dizziness, hypotension, blurred vision, faulty reflexes and perceptions	● Advise the patient to rise slowly, hold on to furniture, and avoid slippery or cluttered floors. ● Warn the patient that the drug may interfere with his driving ability, especially at the beginning of therapy. ● Check the patient's blood pressure in prone and standing positions.
Dry mouth	● Offer the patient mints, ice chips, or chewing gum. ● Advise the patient to hold fluids in the mouth momentarily before swallowing. ● Apply petrolatum to the patient's lips.
Nasal stuffiness	● Add humidity to the room by using a steam vaporizer.
Weight gain	● Encourage the patient to follow a low-calorie diet and to exercise within limits.
Constipation	● Ensure an adequate amount of bulk and fluids in the patient's diet. ● Promote regular exercise. ● Establish regular times for elimination; use a mild laxative, if needed.
Libido changes	● Explain that psychotropic drugs sometimes produce temporary changes in libido. ● Reassure the patient that sexual drive will eventually return to normal.
Photosensitivity, pruritus, grayish purple skin discoloration	● Caution the patient to apply sunscreen and to wear sunglasses and protective clothing when outdoors; direct sunlight intensifies skin rash and discoloration. ● Suggest that the patient use lotion to relieve itching.
Blood dyscrasia (agranulocytosis)	● Teach the patient to report fever, sore throat, unusual malaise, unusual bleeding or bruising, or infection (such as vaginitis, dermatitis, or gastritis). ● Have complete blood count (CBC) and differential studies performed to establish baseline data; then have the studies performed periodically. (If the patient is taking clozapine, weekly CBCs are necessary.) ● Consult the health care provider about decreasing the dosage.
Jaundice or liver damage	● Inform the patient that prolonged treatment or high dosage may decrease liver function. ● Teach the family to observe for yellowish sclera or darkly colored skin. ● Have liver function tests performed occasionally.

Managing the adverse effects of psychotropic drugs *(continued)*

Adverse effects	Nursing interventions
Extrapyramidal reactions (pseudoparkinsonism); akathisia; rigid limbs and drooling; tremors of hands and limbs; taut skin, unsteady gait, and posture changes; akinesia, weakness, fatigue, painful limbs (occurs most commonly in people between ages 15 and 18, in elderly persons, and in women)	• Reduce the dosage, as prescribed; antiparkinsonian drugs may be ordered • Promote safety measures. • Modify care and activities so the patient can maintain self-esteem. • Assist the patient as needed with eating, hygiene, grooming, and mobility.
Tardive dyskinesia (with chronic use of antipsychotics)	• Assess the patient frequently by using the Abnormal Involuntary Movement Scale • Report abnormalities to the prescribing doctor or nurse practitioner.
Neuroleptic malignant syndrome	• Monitor the patient regularly for temperature elevation, vital signs, degree of muscle rigidity, intake and output, and level of consciousness. • Assess the patient's mental status if the temperature rises quickly. • If the patient demonstrates changes in mental status, such as delirium or confusion, notify the prescribing doctor immediately, discontinue the drug, and seek emergency medical treatment. The physician may order bromocriptine (Parlodel) or dantrolene (Dantrium).
Atropinic overload (additive anticholinergic effects)	• Monitor the patient for signs and symptoms of overload including excessive thirst, dry mouth, decreased perspiration, possibility of heat stroke, elevated temperature, red coloration of face, sinus tachycardia, dilated pupils, delirium, and changes in behavior and consciousness. Inform the patient of the signs and symptoms of overload.

◗ Depot preparations are long-acting antipsychotic medications given intramuscularly in an oily preparation that slows the absorption rate; three preparations are available: fluphenazine decanoate, fluphenazine enanthate, and haloperidol

◆ Oral drugs usually are distributed adequately, although food or antacids may decrease their absorption

◆ Drugs are metabolized in the liver and kidneys and excreted through the kidneys, enterohepatic circulation, and feces

◆ Excretion is slow; metabolites may be found in urine up to 6 months after drug discontinuation

■ Adverse effects

◆ Acute dystonic reactions

◗ Muscle spasms of the tongue, face, neck, or back

◗ Possible oculogyric crisis, usually within the first 5 days of treatment

◗ Treatment: antihistamines or anticholinergic drugs

Profile of antipsychotic drugs

Antipsychotic drugs consist of six chemical classes that produce adverse effects of varying intensity. Low-potency drugs tend to exert greater sedative and anticholinergic effects and to cause more postural hypotension. High-potency drugs tend to produce more extrapyramidal adverse effects.

   This chart lists generic and trade names and major effects of representative drugs from each chemical class. (Classes appear in boldface type; subclasses appear in italic type.)

Drug	Adverse effects
Phenothiazines *Aliphatics* chlorpromazine (Thorazine)	• High sedative and hypotensive effects • Medium anticholinergic effect • Low extrapyramidal effects
triflupromazine (Vesprin)	• High sedative and hypotensive effects • Medium anticholinergic and extrapyramidal effects
Piperidines mesoridazine (Serentil) thioridazine (Mellaril)	• Medium sedative, hypotensive, anticholinergic, and extrapyramidal effects • High sedative, hypotensive, and anticholinergic effects • Moderate extrapyramidal effects
Piperazines acetophenazine (Tindal)	• Low sedative, hypotensive, and anticholinergic effects • Medium extrapyramidal effects
fluphenazine (Prolixin)	• Low sedative, hypotensive, and anticholinergic effects • High extrapyramidal effects
perphenazine (Trilafon)	• Low hypotensive and anticholinergic effects • Moderate sedative effects • High extrapyramidal effects
trifluoperazine (Stelazine)	• Medium sedative effects • Low hypotensive and anticholinergic effects • High extrapyramidal effects
Thioxanthene *Piperazine* thiothixene (Navane)	• Low sedative, hypotensive, and anticholinergic effects • High extrapyramidal effects
Dibenzoxazepine loxapine (Loxitane)	• Low hypotensive effect • Medium sedative and anticholinergic effects • Moderate extrapyramidal effects
Butyrophenone haloperidol (Haldol)	• Low sedative, hypotensive, and anticholinergic effects • High extrapyramidal effects
Dihydroindolone molindone (Moban)	• Medium sedative and anticholinergic effects • Low hypotensive effects • Moderate extrapyramidal effects

Profile of antipsychotic drugs *(continued)*

Drug	Adverse effects
Dibenzodiazepine clozapine (Clozaril)	• Low extrapyramidal effects • High (severe) sedative, hypotensive, tachycardia, anticholinergic, and hyper-salivation effects
Benzisoxazole risperidone (Risperdal)	• Low extrapyramidal effects, anxiety, headache, agitation, neuroleptic malignant syndrome

◆ Akathisia
  ▶ Motor restlessness that's commonly mistaken for psychotic restlessness or agitation
  ▶ May appear after the first few days of treatment
  ▶ Symptoms: difficulty in sitting; pacing, fidgeting, constant movement of extremities
  ▶ Treatment: dosage reduction or different medication; sometimes muscle relaxants and anticholinergics are helpful
◆ Pseudoparkinsonism
  ▶ Motor retardation and rigidity
  ▶ Difficulty in initiating or carrying out motor activity
  ▶ Shuffling gait
  ▶ Hypersalivation
  ▶ Tremors in the hands and legs
  ▶ Treatment: anticholinergic medication and dosage reduction
◆ Tardive dyskinesia
  ▶ Potential permanent complication of long-term neuroleptic drug therapy, believed to result from the development of receptors that are supersensitive to dopamine after prolonged blockade
  ▶ Common symptoms
    • Excessive facial movements (including grimacing; blinking; ticlike movements, particularly around the mouth; chewing; and lateral jaw movement)
    • Protrusion of the tongue (sometimes called "fly catcher" tongue), puffing of the cheeks or the tongue in the cheek
    • Thrusting of extremities and neck
    • Involuntary, usually choreoathetoid movements
  ▶ Treatment: dosage reduction or medication discontinuation; because there's no real treatment, prevention is essential
  ▶ Monitor for tardive dyskinesia during drug therapy and after discontinuance

◆ Neuroleptic malignant syndrome
  ▶ Rare, life-threatening reaction to neuroleptic drugs, especially high-potency drugs
  ▶ Causes hyperthermia, rigidity, impaired consciousness, unstable automatic functions, hypertension, hypotension, elevated white blood cell count and creatine kinase level, and cardiac arrhythmias
  ▶ Treatment: immediate discontinuation of the drug, cooling blankets, restoration of hydration and fluid and electrolyte balances, administration of dantrolene sodium and bromocriptine mesylate
◆ Other possible effects
  ▶ Breathing difficulty
  ▶ Uncontrollable hypersalivation
  ▶ Grunting
  ▶ Sedation
  ▶ Hypotension
  ▶ Changes in electrocardiogram (ECG) T waves
  ▶ Lowered seizure threshold
  ▶ Endocrine disturbances
    • Increased prolactin levels from dopamine blockade
    • Amenorrhea
  ▶ Weight gain
  ▶ Changes in libido
  ▶ Photosensitivity
  ▶ Cholestatic hepatitis
  ▶ Blood dyscrasias, including aplastic anemia
  ▶ Anticholinergic effects
    • Dry mouth
    • Blurred vision
    • Constipation
    • Urine retention
  ▶ Treatment: dosage reduction or medication discontinuation
■ Contraindications
  ◆ Known hypersensitivity
  ◆ Comatose states
  ◆ Use in combination with known central nervous system (CNS) depressants, such as alcohol, narcotics, and barbiturates
  ◆ Blood dyscrasias
  ◆ Hepatic, renal, or cardiac dysfunctions
■ Nursing considerations
  ◆ Ensure that the patient undergoes a thorough physiologic and psychological assessment before taking an antipsychotic medication; include family members or significant others in the assessment so they can be informed of drug interactions and potential adverse effects
  ◆ Document all patient and family teaching
  ◆ Encourage the patient to practice sound health habits and to undergo a yearly physical examination

◆ Tell the patient to report adverse reactions or discomfort from the medication

◆ Be aware that safe use during pregnancy hasn't been established; precautions should be taken, particularly during the first trimester

◆ Know that antipsychotic drugs are excreted in breast milk

❖ **Antiparkinsonian drugs**

■ Indication: to relieve the neurologic adverse effects of antipsychotic drugs

■ Mechanism of action: block central cholinergic receptors

■ Absorption, distribution, and elimination (see *Common antiparkinsonian drugs*, page 206)

　◆ Variable absorption in the GI tract

　◆ Cross the blood-brain barrier

　◆ Eliminated in urine and feces

■ Adverse effects

　◆ Anticholinergic

　　▶ Dry mouth

　　▶ Constipation

　　▶ Blurred vision

　　▶ Urine retention

　　▶ Flushed skin

　◆ GI

　　▶ Nausea

　　▶ Vomiting

　◆ Central nervous system

　　▶ Impaired cognitive functioning

　　▶ Disorientation

　　▶ Confusion

　　▶ Hallucinations

　　▶ Restlessness

　　▶ Weakness

　　▶ Drowsiness

　◆ Other

　　▶ Suppression of sweating, causing hyperthermia

　　▶ Toxic psychosis, with symptoms of euphoria, confusion, and disorientation

　　▶ Postural hypotension

■ Contraindications

　◆ Prostatic hypertrophy

　◆ Anuria

　◆ Acute angle-closure glaucoma

■ Nursing considerations

　◆ Teach the patient the proper use of antiparkinsonian drugs; instruct the patient not to increase the dosage without consulting the physician

Common antiparkinsonian drugs

This chart lists the primary effects of the most commonly administered antiparkinsonian drugs.

Drug	Effects
benztropine (Cogentin)	Acts as muscle relaxant, reduces rigidity and drooling, relieves dystonic reactions, exerts sedative actions.
trihexyphenidyl (Artane)	Exerts a mild effect on rigidity and spasms, alleviates tremors; administered during the day for lethargic and akinetic patients.
biperiden (Akineton)	Reduces rigidity and akinesia.
amantadine (Symmetrel)	Improves akathisia, akinesia, dystonias, pseudoparkinsonism, and rigidity; however, tolerance to dosage may develop after 2 to 3 weeks.
diphenhydramine (Benadryl)	Reduces characteristic tremor associated with parkinsonism.

◆ Monitor the patient's intake and output to assess for urine retention (especially in an elderly patient)
◆ Observe the patient for signs of toxicity and additive anticholinergic effects
◆ Administer medications after meals to avoid gastric irritation
◆ Instruct the patient to relieve dry mouth with sugarless gum or candy
◆ Teach the patient to prevent weight gain by avoiding high-calorie drinks and sweets
◆ Be aware of the possible association between use of anticholinergic drugs and minor fetal malformations; if possible, the patient should avoid taking the drug during the first trimester of pregnancy
◆ Caution the patient about breast-feeding while taking these drugs (no supportive data available)

❖ **Tricyclic antidepressants**
■ Indications
    ◆ Depressive disorders
    ◆ Psychotic depression
    ◆ Attention deficit hyperactivity disorder (ADHD)
    ◆ Obsessive-compulsive disorder
    ◆ Organic affective disorder

- ◆ Bulimia
- ◆ Posttraumatic stress disorder
- ◆ Neurogenic pain syndromes
- ◆ Migraine headaches
- ◆ Enuresis in children and adolescents
- ■ Mechanism of action: unknown (drugs may block the reuptake of norepinephrine and serotonin to their presynaptic state, increasing the concentration of these neurotransmitters)
- ■ Absorption, distribution, and elimination (see *Common antidepressant drugs*, page 208)
  - ◆ Absorbed in the GI tract
  - ◆ Binds to plasma and tissue protein
  - ◆ Highly lipophilic, metabolized in the liver, with nonlipophilic metabolites being excreted in feces and urine
- ■ Adverse effects
  - ◆ Allergic: rash
  - ◆ Anticholinergic
    - ▶ Blurred vision
    - ▶ Dry mouth
    - ▶ Constipation
    - ▶ Urine retention
    - ▶ Increased perspiration
    - ▶ Speech difficulty
    - ▶ Mental clouding, confusion, and delirium
  - ◆ Cardiovascular
    - ▶ Postural hypotension
    - ▶ Dizziness
    - ▶ Hypertension
    - ▶ Sinus tachycardia
    - ▶ Premature atrial or ventricular beats
    - ▶ Myocardial depression
    - ▶ Pedal edema
    - ▶ Worsening of heart failure
    - ▶ ECG changes
      - • Depressed ST segment
      - • Flat or inverted T wave
      - • Prolonged QRS complex
  - ◆ GI
    - ▶ Nausea
    - ▶ Vomiting
    - ▶ Heartburn
    - ▶ Weight gain
  - ◆ Neurologic
    - ▶ Drowsiness
    - ▶ Muscle tremors, twitches
    - ▶ Nervousness

Common antidepressant drugs

In treating a patient with depression, the health care provider may prescribe a tricyclic or atypical antidepressant, a monoamine oxidase (MAO) inhibitor, or a selective serotonin reuptake inhibitor. This chart lists commonly administered antidepressants, the intensity of their sedative and anticholinergic effects, and their risk levels for seizure and cardiac toxicity.

Drug	Sedative effects	Anticholinergic effects	Seizure risk	Cardiac toxicity
Tricyclic antidepressants				
amitriptyline (Elavil, Endep)	High	High	Moderate	High
amoxapine (Asendin)	Low	Low	Moderate	Low
desipramine (Norpramin, Pertofrane)	Low	Low	Mild	High
doxepin (Adapin, Sinequan)	High	High	Moderate	High
imipramine (Tofranil, Janimine)	Moderate	High	Moderate	High
maprotiline (Ludiomil)	Moderate	Low	High	Moderate
nortriptyline (Aventyl, Pamelor)	Moderate	Moderate	Mild	Moderate
protriptyline (Vivactil)	Low	Moderate	Moderate	High
trimipramine (Surmontil)	High	Moderate	Moderate	High
Selective serotonin reuptake inhibitors				
bupropion (Wellbutrin)	Low	Low	High	Low
fluoxetine (Prozac)	Low	Low	Low	Low
paroxetine (Paxil)	Low	Moderate	Low	Low
sertraline (Zoloft)	Low	Low	Low	Low
trazodone (Desyrel)	High	Low	Low	Low
venlafaxine (Effexor)	Low	Low	Low	Low
MAO inhibitors				
phenelzine (Nardil)	Low	Low	Low	Low
tranylcypromine (Parnate)	Low	Low	Low	Low

▶ Paresthesia
▶ Fatigue, weakness
▶ Ataxia
▶ Seizures (with overdose or in a patient with a known seizure disorder, hallucinations, delusions, or activation of schizophrenic or manic psychoses)
◆ Overdose and toxicity
▶ Average lethal dose: adults, 30 mg/kg of body weight; children, 20 mg/kg of body weight
▶ Initial symptoms: fever, irritability, confusion, hallucinations, delirium, hypertension, and choreiform movements
▶ Late symptoms: cardiac abnormalities, drowsiness, respiratory depression, cyanosis, heart failure, and shock
▶ Treatment of overdose: hospitalization, with close monitoring of cardiovascular and respiratory systems; removal of drug from the stomach by lavage and administration of activated charcoal

- Contraindications
  - ◆ Excessive use of alcohol and sedatives
  - ◆ History of seizures or suicide attempts
  - ◆ Urine retention
  - ◆ Acute angle-closure glaucoma
  - ◆ Hypersensitivity to the drug
  - ◆ Cardiovascular disease
  - ◆ Concomitant use of monoamine oxidase (MAO) inhibitors (usually)
- Nursing considerations
  - ◆ Teach the patient the proper use of medications, and explain adverse effects
    - ▶ Instruct the patient to take medications at night to prevent daytime drowsiness and dizziness
    - ▶ Reassure the patient that these symptoms will decrease in 2 to 3 weeks
    - ▶ Warn the patient of delayed effects and possible increased suicidal risk after initiating the drug.
  - ◆ Monitor the patient's behavior for early adverse effects of the medications
  - ◆ Observe for increased psychomotor activity
  - ◆ Assess the patient's suicide potential
  - ◆ Instruct the patient to report urine retention
  - ◆ Teach the patient the importance of following a proper diet, with emphasis on increasing roughage and bulk to prevent constipation
  - ◆ Take measures to prevent or minimize dry mouth
    - ▶ Offer sugarless candy and gum
    - ▶ Encourage the patient to increase fluid intake; offer sugarless drinks to prevent weight gain
  - ◆ Know that psychotherapy will be used in conjunction with drug therapy to treat a patient with depression
  - ◆ Be aware that tricyclic antidepressants should be avoided in the first trimester of pregnancy and that they're excreted in breast milk (*Note:* They haven't been proved to have teratogenic effects)

❖ MAO inhibitors

- Indication: symptomatic treatment of depression, especially atypical depression
- Mechanism of action: inhibit the action of the enzyme MAO, thereby preventing the degradation of norepinephrine and serotonin and increasing their concentration in nerve tissue, liver, and lungs
- Absorption, distribution, and elimination
  - ◆ Absorbed in the GI tract
  - ◆ Metabolized in the liver and excreted by the kidneys
- Adverse effects
  - ◆ Anticholinergic (most common)
    - ▶ Blurred vision

- ◗ Dry mouth
- ◗ Constipation
- ◗ Urine retention
- ◗ Increased perspiration
- ◗ Speech difficulty
- ◗ Mental clouding, confusion, and delirium
- ◆ Insomnia and restlessness
- ◆ Hypomania in patients with bipolar disorder
- ◆ Myoclonic jerks during sleep
- ◆ Hypertensive crisis
  - ◗ May occur after the patient ingests food that contains tyramine or takes a drug with sympathomimetic properties (many over-the-counter drugs fit this description)
  - ◗ Can be life-threatening if not treated (discontinuation of the drug; I.V. administration of phentolamine 5 mg, an alpha-receptor antagonist that will lower the patient's blood pressure)
- ■ Contraindications
  - ◆ Kidney or liver disease
  - ◆ Hypertension
  - ◆ Cardiac arrhythmias
  - ◆ Epilepsy
  - ◆ Parkinsonism
- ■ Nursing considerations
  - ◆ Teach the patient the proper use of prescribed medications, and explain their adverse effects
  - ◆ Advise the patient to take these medications early in the day to avoid insomnia
  - ◆ Caution the patient to avoid over-the-counter cold remedies, decongestants (including nasal sprays and drops), antihistamines, sleep aids, stimulants, and appetite suppressants
  - ◆ Instruct the patient to avoid foods that contain high levels of tyramine (aged cheese, meat extracts, pickled herring, sour cream and yogurt, soy sauce, chocolate, dried fruits, sausage, salami, pepperoni, bologna, red wine, beer, sherry, caviar, snails, and fermented foods)
  - ◆ Educate the patient about possible hypotension; demonstrate how to rise slowly from a chair or bed
  - ◆ Urge the patient to report unexpected symptoms, such as headaches and increased palpitations

❖ Antimanic drugs
- ■ Indication: treatment of bipolar disorder
- ■ Mechanism of action: unknown (lithium competes with sodium and other cations, thereby affecting the activity of the nerve cell)
- ■ Absorption, distribution, and elimination
  - ◆ Absorbed in the GI tract

- ◆ Distributed throughout all body tissues, including spinal fluid and breast milk; cross the placental barrier
- ◆ Not metabolized; about 95% excreted in urine
- ■ Adverse effects
  - ◆ GI
    - ❱ Irritation
    - ❱ Nausea
    - ❱ Vomiting
    - ❱ Diarrhea
    - ❱ Thirst
    - ❱ Muscle weakness
    - ❱ Tinnitus
  - ◆ Neurologic
    - ❱ Fine tremor of hand (most common at higher dosages; relieved when medication is discontinued)
    - ❱ Fatigue
    - ❱ Nervousness
  - ◆ Renal: polyuria
  - ◆ Endocrine: hypothyroidism
  - ◆ Toxicity
    - ❱ Mild: can develop gradually over several days
      - • Symptoms: ataxia, confusion, diarrhea, drowsiness, and slurred speech
      - • Treatment: discontinuation of lithium
    - ❱ Severe: can occur when drug levels exceed 1.5 to 2 mEq/liter
      - • Symptom: coma
      - • Treatment: restoration of fluid and electrolyte balance; hemodialysis (more effective) or peritoneal dialysis
      - • Renal toxicity
      - • Goiter
- ■ Contraindications
  - ◆ Cardiovascular disease
  - ◆ Kidney disease
  - ◆ Liver disease
  - ◆ Organic brain damage
  - ◆ Pregnancy
- ■ Nursing considerations
  - ◆ Teach the patient and family the proper use of prescribed medications, and explain interactions and adverse effects
  - ◆ Carefully monitor serum drug levels when the patient begins taking the medication
  - ◆ Observe for signs and symptoms of toxicity
  - ◆ Instruct the patient to report adverse effects of medications
  - ◆ Urge the patient not to self-medicate, particularly with diuretics
  - ◆ Encourage the patient to increase fluid intake (while avoiding drinks with sugar and caffeine)

◆ Instruct the patient to report dietary changes, particularly those involving low-sodium diets

◆ Explain the importance of regular laboratory monitoring (serum drug levels, kidney and thyroid functions, hematology studies)

◆ Remember that congenital defects have been reported with use during pregnancy

◆ Be aware that the drug is excreted in breast milk and that breast-feeding should be discouraged

❖ Benzodiazepines

- ■ Indications
  - ◆ Anxiety
  - ◆ Insomnia
  - ◆ Alcohol withdrawal syndrome
  - ◆ Bipolar disorder, manic phase (in conjunction with lithium)
  - ◆ Seizures
- ■ Mechanism of action: depress the CNS at the limbic system, the brain reticular system, and the cerebral cortex
- ■ Absorption, distribution, and elimination (see *Selected benzodiazepines*)
  - ◗ Well absorbed in the GI tract (although food can delay the rate of absorption)
  - ◗ Distribution and elimination possibly influenced by physical disorders (such as liver disease), smoking, age, and use of other drugs
  - ◗ Found throughout all body tissues and breast milk; cross the placental barrier
  - ◗ Metabolized by the liver and excreted in urine
- ■ Adverse effects
  - ◆ Central nervous system
    - ◗ Depression
    - ◗ Fatigue
    - ◗ Drowsiness
    - ◗ Nystagmus
    - ◗ Muscle weakness
    - ◗ Dysarthria
    - ◗ Ataxia
  - ◆ Anticholinergic
    - ◗ Blurred vision
    - ◗ Confusion
    - ◗ Disorientation (primarily in elderly patients)
  - ◆ Other effects
    - ◗ Paradoxical agitation, rage reactions, insomnia, nightmares, and hallucinations in patients with a history of violent or aggressive behavior
    - ◗ Respiratory depression from high dosages
    - ◗ Toxicity

Selected benzodiazepines

This chart lists the half-life, and primary uses of commonly administered benzodiazepines. Note that half-life and excretion of medications may be prolonged if the patient's liver or kidneys aren't functioning properly.

Drug	Half-life	Primary uses
Short-acting		
triazolam (Halcion)	1.5 to 5.5 hours	Hypnotic
Intermediate		
alprazolam (Xanax)	12 to 15 hours	Antianxiety agent; sedative; treatment of alcohol withdrawal syndrome, depression with anxiety, and panic attacks
halazepam (Paxipam)	14 hours	Antianxiety agent; hypnotic
lorazepam (Ativan)	10 to 20 hours	Antianxiety agent; preoperative sedation; treatment of alcohol withdrawal syndrome, catatonia, and akathisia
oxazepam (Serax)	5 to 20 hours	Antianxiety agent; sedative; treatment of alcohol withdrawal syndrome; reduction of aggression in hostile patients
temazepam (Restoril)	10 to 17 hours	Sedative; hypnotic
Long-acting		
chlordiazepoxide (Librium)	5 to 30 hours	Antianxiety agent; sedative; treatment of alcohol withdrawal syndrome
clonazepam (Klonopin)	18 to 50 hours	Anticonvulsant; antianxiety agent; treatment of panic attacks and akathisia
clorazepate (Tranxene)	30 to 100 hours	Antianxiety agent; treatment of alcohol withdrawal syndrome; adjunct therapy for seizures
diazepam (Valium)	20 to 80 hours	Antianxiety agent; anticonvulsant; muscle relaxant; preoperative sedation; treatment of akathisia
flurazepam (Dalmane)	50 to 100 hours	Hypnotic
prazepam (Centrax)	30 to 100 hours	Antianxiety agent

- Rarely fatal if taken alone
- Can be fatal in combination with other CNS depressants, such as alcohol and barbiturates
- Symptoms of overdose: depressed respirations, hypertension, and coma
- Potential for abuse: patients can build tolerance for benzodiazepines

- Contraindications
  - ◆ Sleep apnea
  - ◆ Liver disease
  - ◆ History of alcohol or drug abuse
- Nursing considerations
  - ◆ Teach the patient the proper use of prescribed medications, and explain their adverse effects
  - ◆ Caution the patient not to use the drug in combination with other CNS depressants, such as alcohol and barbiturates
  - ◆ Warn the patient not to adjust the dosage without consulting the physician, and explain that tolerance may develop with chronic use
  - ◆ Advise the patient to avoid caffeine, which would counteract the effects of the prescribed medication
  - ◆ Caution the patient not to drive a car or operate machinery while taking the medication because mental alertness may be impaired
  - ◆ Continue to assess the patient's response to the medication
    - ▶ Determine if target symptoms are being treated
    - ▶ Assess whether oversedation has occurred (particularly with an elderly patient)
  - ◆ Warn the patient that antianxiety agents can aggravate symptoms of depression.

❖ Sedative-hypnotics

- Indications
  - ◆ Anxiety (barbiturates are seldom used as antianxiety agents because of their potential for tolerance, dependence, and toxicity; antihistamines are sometimes used as antianxiety agents in pediatric and elderly patients)
  - ◆ Insomnia (chloral hydrate derivatives)
  - ◆ Prevention of alcohol withdrawal symptoms (chloral hydrate derivatives)
- Mechanism of action
  - ◆ Barbiturates: suppress the reticular activating formation of the midbrain, resulting in sedation, sleep, and anesthesia
  - ◆ Antihistamines: compete with histamine for histamine receptor sites on effector cells
  - ◆ Chloral hydrate derivatives: not fully understood
- Absorption, distribution, and elimination (see *Selected sedative-hypnotics*)
  - ◆ Barbiturates: absorbed in the GI tract; metabolized in the liver; excreted in urine
  - ◆ Antihistamines: absorbed in the GI tract but only 40% to 60% enters the systemic circulation; metabolized in the liver; excreted in urine
  - ◆ Chloral hydrate derivatives: absorbed in the GI tract or rectal mucosa; metabolized in the liver; excreted by the kidneys and through bile in feces

Selected sedative-hypnotics

This chart lists the half-life, and primary uses of commonly prescribed sedative-hypnotics.

Drug	Half-life	Primary uses
Antihistamines		
diphenhydramine (Benadryl)	3 to 4 hours	Hypnotic; antianxiety agent
doxylamine (Unisom)	10 hours	Hypnotic
hydroxyzine (Atarax)	3 hours	Antianxiety agent; hypnotic; sedative
Barbiturates		
amobarbital (Amytal)	20 hours	Hypnotic; also used as a diagnostic aid in hysteria
pentobarbital (Nembutal)	35 to 50 hours	Hypnotic; preoperative sedation
secobarbital (Seconal)	35 to 50 hours	Hypnotic; preoperative sedation
Chloral hydrate derivatives		
chloral hydrate (Noctec)	8 to 10 hours	Hypnotic

■ Adverse effects
  ◆ Barbiturates
    ▸ Dependence with long-term use
    ▸ Symptoms of toxicity with long-term use
      • Excitement
      • Restlessness
      • Delirium
      • Ataxia
      • Nystagmus
      • Stupor
      • Hypothermia
  ◆ Antihistamines
    ▸ Delirium
    ▸ Confusion
    ▸ Orthostatic hypotension
    ▸ Urine retention
  ◆ Chloral hydrate derivatives
    ▸ Dependence with use after several weeks
    ▸ Symptoms of toxicity with long-term use
      • Incoordination
      • Slurred speech
      • Fatigue
      • Tremors
      • Possible coma, respiratory depression, and cardiac dysfunction
■ Contraindications
  ◆ Previous addiction

◆ Liver or kidney impairment
◆ Respiratory disease
◆ Hypersensitivity
■ Nursing considerations
◆ Teach the patient the proper use of prescribed medications, and explain their adverse effects
◆ Warn the patient not to adjust the dosage without consulting the physician
◆ Caution the patient about the potential for tolerance and dependence with chronic use
◆ Inform the patient that continued use may worsen sleep patterns
◆ Suggest alternative methods of treating insomnia
▶ Avoid caffeine if possible during the day and particularly after 6 p.m.
▶ Drink herbal teas
◆ Encourage the patient to refrain from daytime naps and to follow a daily routine that incorporates exercise and relaxation techniques
◆ Warn the patient about the potential for increased tolerance and possibility of dependence.

Review questions

1. A patient is prescribed haloperidol (Haldol). The nurse should instruct the patient to:

○ **A.** use a sunscreen because the drug increases photosensitivity.

○ **B.** take the medication with food.

○ **C.** maintain therapeutic blood levels.

○ **D.** abstain from eating aged cheese.

Correct answer: A Antipsychotics such as haloperidol increase the patient's sensitivity to the sun. Options B, C, and D aren't appropriate instructions for taking this drug.

2. A patient may abuse or develop a dependency on which of the following drugs?

○ **A.** Lithium (Eskalith) and valproic acid (Depakote)

○ **B.** Verapamil (Calan) and chlorpromazine (Thorazine)

○ **C.** Alprazolam (Xanax) and pentobarbital (Nembutal)

○ **D.** Clozapine (Clozaril) and amitriptyline (Elavil)

Correct answer: C Long-term use of benzodiazepines, such as alprazolam, or barbiturates, such as pentobarbital may increase a patient's tolerance for the drug. Increased tolerance can lead to drug dependency or abuse. Lithium, valproic acid, verapamil, chlorpromazine, clozapine, and amitriptyline aren't associated with dependency or abuse.

3. Which of the following instructions should the nurse incorporate into her teaching plan for a patient taking chlordiazepoxide (Librium)?

○ **A.** Don't mix chlordiazepoxide with other CNS depressants or alcohol.

○ **B.** Don't take chlordiazepoxide before going to sleep.

○ **C.** Don't take chlordiazepoxide on an empty stomach.

○ **D.** Don't combine chlordiazepoxide with aged cheese.

Correct answer: A Antianxiety agents such as chlordiazepoxide potentiate the action of other CNS depressants, which can result in an accidental overdose. Chlodiazepoxide can be taken before going to sleep or on an empty stomach. Aged cheese has no effect on chlordiazepoxide.

4. Antiparkinsonian drugs can be indicated for which of the following?

○ **A.** Symptomatic treatment of depression

○ **B.** To relieve the neurologic adverse effects of antipsychotic drugs

○ **C.** Treatment of bipolar disorder

○ **D.** Treatment of alcohol withdrawal syndrome

Correct answer: B Antiparkinsonian drugs can be indicated to help relieve the neurologic adverse effects of antipsychotic drugs. MAO inhibitors are indicated for symptomatic treatment of depression. Antimanic drugs are used to treat bipolar disorder. Bezodiazepines help to treat alcohol withdrawal syndrome.

5. An elderly patient who takes lithium daily tells the nurse that she's feeling nauseous and has diarrhea. The nurse suspects that the patient is experiencing lithium toxicity. The nurse should also determine if the patient has:

○ **A.** ataxia.

○ **B.** a fever.

○ **C.** missed taking the drug for a few days.

○ **D.** been able to keep her medicine down

Correct answer: A Signs and symptoms of lithium toxicity include diarrhea, nausea, and ataxia. A patient who has missed a few doses of lithium wouldn't exhibit these signs and symptoms. Fever may be caused by dehydration, not lithium toxicity.

Appendices, Posttest, and Index

Appendix A
Standards of psychiatric and mental health clinical nursing practice

In 1973, the American Nurses Association issued standards to improve the quality of care provided by psychiatric and mental health nurses. These standards, last revised in 2000, apply to generalists and specialists working in any setting in which psychiatric and mental health nursing is practiced (standards Vh through Vj apply to the advanced practice registered nurse in psychiatric and mental health [APRN-PMH] specialist only). Listed here are the standards of care and standards of professional performance, along with their rationales and measurement criteria.

Standards of care

Standards of care pertain to professional nursing activities that are demonstrated by the nurse through the nursing process. These involve assessment, diagnosis, outcome identification, planning, implementation, and evaluation. The nursing process is the foundation of clinical decision making and encompasses all significant action taken by nurses in providing psychiatric and mental health care to all patients.

STANDARD I. ASSESSMENT

The psychiatric and mental health nurse collects patient health data.

Rationale

The assessment interview—which requires linguistically and culturally effective communication skills, interviewing, behavioral observation, database record review, and comprehensive assessment of the patient and relevant systems—enables the psychiatric and mental health nurse to make sound clinical judgments and plan appropriate interventions with the patient.

Measurement criteria

1. The priority of data collection is determined by the patient's immediate condition or need.
2. The data may include but are not limited to:
   a. ability to remain safe and not be in danger of oneself and others
   b. patient's central complaint, symptoms, or focus of concern

   c. physical, developmental, cognitive, mental, and emotional health status

   d. demographic profile and history of health patterns and illness

   e. family, social, cultural, and community systems

   f. daily activities, functional health status, substance use, health habits, and social roles, including work and sexual functioning

   g. interpersonal relationships, communication skills, and coping patterns

   h. spiritual, religious, or philosophical beliefs and values

   i. economic, political, legal, and environmental factors affecting health

   j. significant support systems, both available and underutilized

   k. health beliefs and practices

   l. knowledge, satisfaction, and motivation to change, related to health

   m. strengths and competencies that can be used to promote health

   n. current and past medications, including prescribed and over-the-counter

   o. medication interactions and history of adverse effects

   p. complementary therapies used to promote health and treat mental illness

   q. other contributing factors that influence health.

3. Pertinent data are collected from multiple sources using various assessment techniques and standardized instruments as appropriate. Multiple sources of assessment data can include not only the patient, but also the family, social network, other health care providers, past and current medical records, and community agencies and systems (with consideration of the patient's confidentiality).

4. The patient, family and significant others, and interdisciplinary team members are involved in the assessment process and data analysis.

5. The patient as well as family and significant others are informed of their respective roles and responsibilities in the assessment process and data analysis.

6. The assessment process is systematic and ongoing.

7. The data collection is based on clinical judgment to ensure that relevant and necessary data are collected.

8. The database is synthesized, prioritized, and documented in a retrievable form.

STANDARD II. DIAGNOSIS

The psychiatric and mental health nurse analyzes the assessment data in determining diagnoses.

Rationale

The basis for providing psychiatric and mental health nursing care is the recognition and identification of patterns of response to actual or potential psychiatric illnesses, mental health problems, and potential comorbid physical illnesses.

Measurement criteria

1. Diagnoses and potential problem statements are derived from assessment data.
2. Interpersonal, systemic, or environmental circumstances that affect the mental well-being of the individual, family, or community are identified.
3. The diagnosis is based on an accepted framework that supports the psychiatric and mental health nursing knowledge and judgment used in analyzing the data.
4. Diagnoses conform to accepted classifications systems—such as North American Nursing Diagnosis Association (NANDA) Nursing Diagnosis Classification, International Classification of Diseases and Statistical Manual of Mental Diseases (WHO, 1993), and the *Diagnostic and Statistical Manual of Mental Disorders*, 4th Edition, Text Revision (APA, 2000) used in the practice setting.
5. Diagnoses and risk factors are validated with the patient, family and significant others, and other health care providers when appropriate and possible.
6. Diagnoses identify actual or potential psychiatric illness and mental health problems of patients.
7. Diagnoses and clinical impressions are documented in a manner that facilitates identification of patient outcomes and their use in the plan of care and research.

STANDARD III. OUTCOME IDENTIFICATION

The psychiatric and mental health nurse identifies expected outcomes individualized for the patient.

Rationale

Within the context of providing nursing care, the ultimate goal is to influence health outcomes and improve the patient's health status.

Measurement criteria

1. Expected outcomes are derived from the diagnoses.
2. Expected outcomes are patient-oriented, therapeutically sound, realistic, attainable, and cost-effective.
3. Expected outcomes are documented as measurable goals using standard classifications when available.
4. Expected outcomes are formulated by the nurse and the patient, family and significant others, and interdisciplinary team members, when possible.
5. Expected outcomes are realistic in relation to the patient's present and potential capabilities and quality of life.
6. Expected outcomes are identified with consideration of the associated benefits and costs.
7. Expected outcomes estimate a time for attainment.
8. Expected outcomes provide direction for continuity of care.

9. Expected outcomes reflect current scientific knowledge in mental health care.

10. Expected outcomes serve as a record of change in the patient's health status.

STANDARD IV. PLANNING

The psychiatric and mental health nurse develops a plan of care that is negotiated among the patient, nurse, family and significant others, and health care team, and that prescribes evidence-based interventions to attain expected outcomes.

Rationale

A plan of care is used to guide therapeutic intervention, systematically document progress, and achieve the expected patient outcomes.

Measurement criteria

1. The plan is individualized, according to the patient's characteristics, mental health problems, and condition, and:

   a. identifies priorities of care in relation to expected outcomes

   b. identifies effective interventions to achieve the outcomes

   c. specifies interventions that reflect current psychiatric and mental health nursing practice and research

   d. reflects the patient's motivation, health beliefs, and functional capabilities

   e. includes an education program related to the patient's health problems, stress management, treatment regimen, relapse prevention, self-care activities, and quality of life

   f. indicates responsibilities of the nurse, the patient, the family and significant others, and the interdisciplinary team members in implementing the plan

   g. gives direction to patient-care activities — designated by the nurse — to the family, significant others, and other care clinicians

   h. provides for appropriate referral and case management to ensure continuity of care

   i. considers the benefits and costs of interventions in relation to outcomes.

2. The plan is developed in collaboration with the patient, family and significant others, and interdisciplinary team members, when appropriate.

3. The plan is documented in a format that allows modification as necessary, interdisciplinary access to its information, and retrieval of data for analysis and research.

STANDARD V. IMPLEMENTATION

The psychiatric and mental health nurse implements the interventions identified in the plan of care.

Rationale

In implementing the plan of care, psychiatric and mental health nurses use a wide range of interventions designed to prevent mental and physical illness and to promote, maintain, and restore mental and physical health. Psychiatric and mental health nurses select interventions according to their level of practice. At the basic level, the nurse may select counseling, milieu therapy, self-care activities, psychobiological interventions, health teaching, case management, health promotion and health maintenance, crisis intervention, community-based care, psychiatric home health care, telehealth, and a variety of other approaches to meet the mental health needs of the patient. In addition to the intervention options available to the basic-level psychiatric and mental health nurse, at the advanced level, the APRN-PMH may provide consultation, engage in psychotherapy, and prescribe pharmacologic agents where permitted by state statutes or regulations.

Measurement criteria

1. A therapeutic nurse-patient relationship is established and maintained throughout treatment.
2. Interventions are based on research when available.
3. Interventions are implemented according to the established plan of care.
4. Interventions are performed according to the psychiatric and mental health nurse's level of education and practice.
5. Interventions are performed in a safe, timely, ethical, and appropriate manner.
6. Interventions are modified based on continued assessment of the patient's response to treatment and other clinical indicators of effectiveness.
7. Interventions are documented in a format that is related to patient outcomes, accessible to the interdisciplinary team, and retrievable for future data analysis and research.

STANDARD Va. COUNSELING

The psychiatric and mental health nurse uses counseling interventions to assist patients in improving or regaining their previous coping abilities, fostering mental health and preventing mental illness and disability.

Measurement criteria

1. Counseling promotes the patient's personal and social integration.
2. Counseling reinforces healthy behaviors and interaction patterns and helps the patient modify or discontinue unhealthy ones.
3. The documentation of counseling interventions—including communication and interviewing techniques, problem-solving skills, crisis intervention, stress management, relaxation techniques, assertiveness training, conflict resolution, and behavior modification—is completed in a timely manner.

STANDARD Vb. MILIEU THERAPY

The psychiatric and mental health nurse provides, structures, and maintains a therapeutic environment in collaboration with the patient and other health care providers.

Measurement criteria

1. The patient is familiarized with the physical environment, the schedule of activities, and the norms and rules that govern behavior and activities of daily living, as applicable.
2. Current knowledge of the effects of the patient's environment on the patient is used to guide nursing actions and provide a safe environment.
3. The therapeutic environment is designed utilizing the physical environment, social structures, culture, and other available resources.
4. Therapeutic communication among patients and staff supports an effective milieu.
5. Specific activities are selected that meet the patient's physical and mental health needs.
6. Limits of any kind (for example, restriction of privileges, restraint, seclusion, timeout) are used in a humane manner, are the least restrictive necessary, and are employed only as long as needed to ensure the safety of the patient and of others.
7. The patient is given information about the need for limits and the conditions necessary for removal of the restriction, as appropriate.

STANDARD Vc. PROMOTION OF SELF-CARE ACTIVITIES

The psychiatric and mental health nurse structures interventions around the patient's activities of daily living to foster self-care and mental and physical well-being.

Measurement criteria

1. The self-care activities chosen are appropriate for the patient's physical and mental status, as well as age, developmental level, gender, social orientation, ethnic and social background, and education.
2. The self-care interventions assist the patient in assuming personal responsibility for activities of daily living, including maintaining a medical regimen, engaging in health-promoting behaviors, and seeking therapeutic interventions when appropriate.
3. Self-care interventions are aimed at maintaining and improving the patient's functional status and quality of life.

STANDARD Vd. PSYCHOBIOLOGICAL INTERVENTIONS

The psychiatric and mental health nurse uses knowledge of psychobiological interventions and applies clinical skills to restore the patient's health and prevent further disability.

Measurement criteria

1. Current research findings are applied to guide nursing actions related to psychopharmacology, other psychobiological therapies, and complementary therapies.
2. Psychopharmacologic agents' intended actions, untoward or interactive effects, and therapeutic doses are monitored, as are blood levels, vital signs, and laboratory values where appropriate.
3. Nursing interventions are directed toward alleviating untoward effects of psychobiological interventions, when possible.
4. Nursing observations about the patient's response to psychobiological interventions are communicated to other health clinicians.

STANDARD Ve. HEALTH TEACHING

The psychiatric and mental health nurse, through health teaching, assists patients in achieving satisfying, productive, and healthy patterns of living.

Measurement criteria

1. Health teaching is based on principles of learning.
2. Health teaching occurs on an individual basis or within a group context, depending on information content and patient ability.
3. Health teaching includes information about coping, interpersonal relations, mental health problems, mental disorders, and treatments and their effects on daily living, as well as information pertinent to physical status or developmental needs.
4. Constructive feedback and positive rewards reinforce the patient's learning.
5. Practice sessions and experiential learning are used as needed.
6. Health teaching provides opportunities for the patient as well as family and significant others to question, discuss, and explore their thoughts and feelings about past, current, and projected use of therapies and to make informed choices.

STANDARD Vf. CASE MANAGEMENT

The psychiatric and mental health nurse provides case management to coordinate comprehensive health services and ensure continuity of care.

Measurement criteria

1. Case management services are based on a comprehensive approach to the patient's physical, mental, emotional, and social health problems, as well as resource availability.
2. Case management services are provided in terms of the patient's needs and resources and the accessibility, availability, quality, and cost-effectiveness of care.
3. Health-related services and more specialized care are negotiated on behalf of the patient with the appropriate agencies and providers as needed.
4. Relationships with agencies and providers are maintained throughout the patient's use of the health care services to ensure continuity of care.

STANDARD Vg. HEALTH PROMOTION AND HEALTH MAINTENANCE

The psychiatric and mental health nurse employs strategies and interventions to promote and maintain mental health and prevent mental illness.

Measurement criteria

1. Health promotion and disease prevention strategies are based on knowledge of health beliefs, practices, evidence-based findings, and epidemiologic principles, together with the social, cultural, and political issues that affect mental health in an identified community.

2. Health promotion and disease prevention interventions are designed for patients identified as at-risk for mental health problems.

3. Consumer alliances and participation are encouraged in identifying mental health problems in the community and in planning, implementing, and evaluating programs to address those problems.

4. Community resources are identified to assist consumers in using prevention and mental health care services appropriately.

5. Research findings are utilized to promote health and prevent mental illness.

Advanced practice interventions

The following interventions (Vh-Vj) may only be performed by the APRN-PMH.

STANDARD Vh. PSYCHOTHERAPY

The APRN-PMH uses individual, group, and family psychotherapy and other therapeutic treatments to assist patients in preventing mental illness and disability, treating mental health disorders, and improving mental-health status and functional abilities.

Measurement criteria

1. The therapeutic contract with the patient is structured to include:
    a. purpose, goals, and expected outcomes
    b. time, place, and frequency of therapy
    c. participants involved in therapy
    d. confidentiality
    e. availability and means of contacting therapist
    f. responsibilities of both patient and therapist
    g. fees and payment schedule.

2. Knowledge of personality theory, growth and development, psychology, psychopathology, social systems, small-group and family dynamics, stress and adaptation, and theories related to selected therapeutic methods is used, based on the patient's needs.

3. Therapeutic principles are used to understand and interpret the patient's emotions, thoughts, and behaviors.

4. The patient is helped to deal constructively with thoughts, emotions, and behaviors.

5. Increasing responsibility and independence are fostered in the patient to reinforce healthy behaviors and interactions.

6. In the therapist's absence, provision for care is arranged.

7. When it is determined that the provision of some aspect of physical care required by the patient would impair the therapist-patient relationship, referral for that care is made to another clinician.

STANDARD Vi. PRESCRIPTIVE AUTHORITY AND TREATMENT

The APRN-PMH uses prescriptive authority, procedures, and treatments in accordance with state and federal laws and regulations to treat symptoms of psychiatric illness and improve functional health status.

Measurement criteria

1. Psychiatric treatment interventions and procedures are evidence-based and are prescribed according to the patient's mental health care needs.

2. Procedures are used as needed in the delivery of comprehensive care.

3. Psychopharmacological agents are prescribed based on a knowledge of psychopathology, neurobiology, physiology, expected therapeutic actions, anticipated adverse effects, and courses of action for unintended or toxic effects.

4. Pharmacologic agents are prescribed based on clinical indicators of the patient's status, including the results of diagnostic and laboratory tests, as appropriate.

5. Intended effects and potential adverse effects of pharmacologic and nonpharmacologic treatments are monitored and treated as necessary.

6. Information about intended effects, potential adverse effects of the proposed prescription, and other treatment options, including no treatment, is provided to the patient.

7. Informed consent is obtained for treatment.

STANDARD Vj. CONSULTATION

The APRN-PMH provides consultation to enhance the abilities of other clinicians, to provide services for patients, and to effect change in the system.

Measurement criteria

1. Consultation activities are based on models of consultation, systems principles, communication and interviewing techniques, problem-solving skills, change theories, and other theories as indicated.

2. Consultation is initiated at the request of the consultee.

3. A working alliance, based on mutual respect and role responsibilities, is established with the patient or consultee.

4. Consultation recommendations are communicated in terms that facilitate understanding and involve the consultee in decision making.

5. Implementation of the system change or plan of care remains the consultee's responsibility.

STANDARD VI. EVALUATION

The psychiatric and mental health nurse evaluates the patient's progress in attaining expected outcomes.

Rationale

Nursing care is a dynamic process involving change in the patient's health status over time, giving rise to the need for new data, different diagnoses, and modifications in the plan of care. Therefore, evaluation is a continuous process of appraising the effect of nursing and treatment regimens on the patient's health status and expected outcomes.

Measurement criteria

1. Evaluation is systematic, ongoing, and criterion-based.
2. The patient, family or significant others, and other health care clinicians are involved in the evaluation process, as possible, to ascertain the patient's level of satisfaction with care and evaluate the cost and benefits associated with the treatment process.
3. The effectiveness of interventions in relation to outcomes is evaluated, using standardized methods as appropriate.
4. The patient's responses to treatment are documented in a format that is related to expected outcomes, accessible to the interdisciplinary team, and retrievable for data analysis and future research.
5. Ongoing assessment data are used to revise diagnoses, outcomes, and the plan of care as needed.
6. Revisions in the diagnoses, outcomes, and the plan of care are documented.
7. The revised plan provides for continuity of care.

Standards of professional performance

Standards of professional performance describe a competent level of behavior in the professional role, including activities related to quality of care, performance appraisal, education, collegiality, ethics, collaboration, research, and resource utilization. All psychiatric and mental health nurses are expected to engage in professional role activities appropriate to their education, position, and practice setting. Therefore, some standards or measurement criteria identify these activities.

While standards of professional performance describe the roles of all professional nurses, many other responsibilities are hallmarks of psychiatric and mental health nursing. These nurses should be self-directed and purposeful in seeking necessary knowledge and skills to enhance career goals. Other activities—such as membership in professional organizations, certification in specialty or advanced practice, continuing education, and further academic education—are desirable methods of enhancing the psychiatric and mental health nurse's professionalism.

STANDARD I. QUALITY OF CARE

The psychiatric and mental health nurse systematically evaluates the quality of care and effectiveness of psychiatric and mental health nursing practice.

Rationale

The dynamic nature of the mental health care environment and the growing body of psychiatric nursing knowledge and research provide the impetus and the means for the psychiatric and mental health nurse to be competent in clinical practice, to continue to develop professionally, and to improve the quality of patient care.

Measurement criteria

1. The psychiatric and mental health nurse participates in quality-of-care activities as appropriate to the nurse's position, education, and practice environment. Such activities can include:

a. identification of aspects of care important for quality monitoring—for example, functional status, symptom management and control, health behaviors and practices, safety, patient satisfaction, and quality of life

b. utilization of existing, or development of new, quality indicators used to monitor the effectiveness of psychiatric and mental health nursing care

c. collection of data to monitor quality and effectiveness of psychiatric and mental health nursing care

d. analysis of quality data to identify opportunities for improving psychiatric and mental health nursing care

e. formulation of recommendations to improve psychiatric and mental health nursing practice or patient outcomes

f. implementation of activities to enhance the quality of psychiatric and mental health nursing practice

g. participation on interdisciplinary teams that evaluate clinical practice or mental health services

h. development of policies and procedures to improve quality psychiatric and mental health care.

2. The psychiatric and mental health nurse seeks feedback from the patient as well as family and significant others about quality and outcomes of the patient's care.

3. The psychiatric and mental health nurse uses the results of quality-of-care activities to initiate changes throughout the mental health care delivery system, as appropriate.

STANDARD II. PERFORMANCE APPRAISAL

The psychiatric and mental health nurse evaluates one's own psychiatric and mental health nursing practice in relation to professional practice standards and relevant statutes and regulations.

Rationale

The psychiatric and mental health nurse is accountable to the public for providing competent clinical care and has an inherent responsibility as a professional to evaluate the role and performance of psychiatric and mental health nursing practice according to standards established by the profession.

Measurement criteria

1. The psychiatric and mental health nurse engages in performance appraisal of one's own clinical practice and role performance with peers or supervisors on a regular basis, identifying areas of strength as well as areas for professional and practice development.
2. The psychiatric and mental health nurse seeks constructive feedback regarding one's own practice and role performance from peers, professional colleagues, patients, and others.
3. The psychiatric and mental health nurse takes action to achieve goals identified during performance appraisal and peer review, resulting in changes in practice and role performance.
4. The psychiatric and mental health nurse participates in peer review activities when possible.
5. The nurse's practice reflects knowledge of current professional practice standards, laws, and regulations.

STANDARD III. EDUCATION

The psychiatric and mental health nurse acquires and maintains current knowledge in nursing practice.

Rationale

The rapid expansion of knowledge pertaining to basic and behavioral sciences, technology, information systems, and research requires a commitment to learning throughout the psychiatric and mental health nurse's professional career. Formal education, continuing education, independent learning activities, and experiential and other learning activities are some of the means the psychiatric and mental health nurse can use to enhance nursing expertise and advance the profession.

Measurement criteria

1. The psychiatric and mental health nurse participates in professional development activities to improve clinical knowledge, enhance role performance, and increase knowledge of professional issues.
2. The psychiatric and mental health nurse seeks experiences and independent learning activities to maintain and develop clinical skills.
3. The psychiatric and mental health nurse seeks additional knowledge and skills appropriate to the practice setting by participating in educational programs and activities, conferences, workshops, and interdisciplinary professional meetings.

4. The psychiatric and mental health nurse documents one's own educational activities.

5. The APRN-PMH maintains a mechanism for ongoing clinical supervision of practice.

STANDARD IV. COLLEGIALITY

The psychiatric and mental health nurse interacts with and contributes to the professional development of peers, health care clinicians, and others as colleagues.

Rationale

The psychiatric and mental health nurse is responsible for sharing knowledge, research, and clinical information with colleagues, through formal and informal teaching methods, to enhance professional growth.

Measurement criteria

1. The psychiatric and mental health nurse uses opportunities in practice to exchange knowledge, skills, and clinical observations with colleagues and others.

2. The psychiatric and mental health nurse assists others in identifying teaching and learning needs related to clinical care, role performance, and professional development.

3. The psychiatric and mental health nurse provides peers with constructive feedback regarding their practices.

4. The psychiatric and mental health nurse contributes to an environment that is conducive to education of nursing students, other health care students, and others, as appropriate.

5. The psychiatric and mental health nurse actively promotes interdisciplinary collaboration.

6. The psychiatric and mental health nurse contributes to a supportive and healthy work environment.

STANDARD V. ETHICS

The psychiatric and mental health nurse's assessments, actions, and recommendations on behalf of patients are determined and implemented in an ethical manner.

Rationale

The public's trust and its right to humane psychiatric and mental health care are upheld by professional nursing practice. Ethical standards describe a code of behaviors to guide professional practice. People with psychiatric and mental health needs are a vulnerable population. The foundation of psychiatric and mental health nursing practice is the development of a therapeutic relationship with the patient. Boundaries need to be established to safeguard the patient's well-being.

Measurement criteria

1. The psychiatric and mental health nurse's practice is guided by the *ANA Code for Nurses.*

2. The psychiatric and mental health nurse establishes appropriate boundaries and maintains a therapeutic and professional relationship with patients at all times.

3. The psychiatric and mental health nurse maintains patient confidentiality within ethical, legal, and regulatory parameters.

4. The psychiatric and mental health nurse functions as a patient advocate.

5. The psychiatric and mental health nurse monitors any personal biases and seeks consultation or supervision as needed to deliver care in a nonjudgmental and nondiscriminatory manner sensitive to patient diversity.

6. The psychiatric and mental health nurse seeks to prevent ethical problems, identifies ethical dilemmas that occur within the practice environment, and seeks available resources to help resolve ethical dilemmas.

7. The psychiatric and mental health nurse reports abuse of patients' rights and incompetent, unethical, and illegal practices.

8. The psychiatric and mental health nurse participates in the informed consent process (including the right to refuse) for patient's procedures, tests, treatments, and research participation, as appropriate.

9. The psychiatric and mental health nurse carefully monitors and manages self-disclosure in a therapeutic relationship.

10. The psychiatric and mental health nurse doesn't promote or engage in intimate sexual or business relationships with current or former patients, and recognizes that to engage in such a relationship is unusual and an exception.

11. The psychiatric and mental health nurse guards against exploitation of information furnished by the patient.

12. The psychiatric and mental health nurse is aware of and avoids the dangers of using the power inherent in the therapeutic relationship to influence the patient in ways not related to the treatment goals.

STANDARD VI. COLLABORATION

The psychiatric and mental health nurse collaborates with the patient, family and significant others, and health care clinicians in providing care.

Rationale

Psychiatric and mental health nursing practice requires a coordinated, ongoing interaction between consumers and providers to deliver comprehensive services to the patient and the community. Through the collaborative process, different abilities of health care clinicians are used to identify problems; communicate, plan, and implement interventions; and evaluate mental health services.

Measurement criteria

1. The psychiatric and mental health nurse collaborates with the patient, family and significant others, and health care clinicians in the formulation of overall goals, plans, and decisions related to patient care and the delivery of mental health services.
2. The psychiatric and mental health nurse consults with other health care clinicians on patient care, as appropriate.
3. The psychiatric and mental health nurse makes referrals, including provisions for continuity of care as needed.
4. The psychiatric and mental health nurse collaborates with other disciplines in teaching, consultation, management, and research activities.

STANDARD VII. RESEARCH

The psychiatric and mental health nurse contributes to the nursing and mental health field through the use of research.

Rationale

Nurses in psychiatric and mental health nursing are responsible for contributing to the further development of the field of mental health by participating in research. At the basic level of practice, the psychiatric and mental health nurse uses research findings to improve clinical care and identifies clinical problems for research study. At the advanced level, the psychiatric and mental health nurse engages and collaborates with others in the research process to discover, examine, and test knowledge, theories, and creative approaches to practice.

Measurement criteria

1. The psychiatric and mental health nurse uses the best available evidence, preferably health-related research data, to develop a plan of care, interventions, and expected outcomes.
2. The psychiatric and mental health nurse participates in research as appropriate given the nurse's position, education, and practice environment. Such activities may include:

   a. identification of clinical problems suitable for psychiatric and mental health nursing research

   b. participation in data collection

   c. participation in a unit, organization, or community research committee or program

   d. sharing research findings with others through discussion groups, professional presentations, and publications

   e. conducting research as an individual investigator or as a member of a research team according to education and experience

   f. critiquing research for application to practice

   g. using research findings in the development of policies, procedures, and practice guidelines for patient care

   h. consulting with research colleagues and experts.

3. The psychiatric and mental health nurse participates in clinical trials and human-subject protection activities as appropriate, recognizing the needs of the vulnerable subjects in the research study.

STANDARD VIII. RESOURCE UTILIZATION

The psychiatric and mental health nurse considers factors related to safety, effectiveness, and cost in planning and delivering patient care.

Rationale

The patient is entitled to psychiatric and mental health care that is safe, effective, and affordable. As the cost of health care increases, treatment decisions must be made in such a way as to maximize resources that maintain quality of care. The psychiatric and mental health nurse seeks to provide cost-effective quality care by using the most appropriate resources and delegating care to the most appropriate, qualified health care clinician.

Measurement criteria

1. The psychiatric and mental health nurse evaluates factors related to safety, effectiveness, availability, and cost when choosing between two or more practice options that result in the same expected patient outcome.
2. The psychiatric and mental health nurse assists the patient and family or significant others in identifying and securing appropriate and available services that address mental health needs.
3. The psychiatric and mental health nurse refers, assigns, or delegates case activities as defined by the state practice acts and according to the knowledge and skills of the designated caregiver.
4. If the psychiatric and mental health nurse refers, assigns, or delegates case activities, it is based on the mental health needs and conditions of the patient, the potential for harm, the stability of the patient's condition, the complexity of the task, and the predictability of the outcome.
5. The psychiatric and mental health nurse assists the patient, family, and significant others in becoming informed consumers about the benefits, risks, and costs of mental health treatment and care.
6. The psychiatric and mental health nurse documents the effects of resource utilization and changing patterns of mental health care delivery on psychiatric and mental health nursing and patient outcomes.

Adapted from: *Scope and Standards of Psychiatric and Mental Health Nursing Practice*. Washington D.C.: American Nurses Association, 2000, with permission of the publisher.

Appendix B
NANDA Taxonomy II

The North American Nursing Diagnosis Association (NANDA) endorsed its first nursing diagnosis taxonomic structure, NANDA Taxonomy I, in 1986. This taxonomy has been revised several times, most recently in 2000. The new Taxonomy II has a code structure that's compliant with the recommendations of the National Library of Medicine concerning health care terminology codes. The taxonomy that appears here represents the accepted classification system for nursing diagnosis.

Taxonomy II code	Nursing diagnosis
00001	Imbalanced nutrition: More than body requirements
00002	Imbalanced nutrition: Less than body requirements
00003	Risk for imbalanced nutrition: More than body requirements
00004	Risk for infection
00005	Risk for imbalanced body temperature
00006	Hypothermia
00007	Hyperthermia
00008	Ineffective thermoregulation
00009	Autonomic dysreflexia
00010	Risk for autonomic dysreflexia
00011	Constipation
00012	Perceived constipation
00013	Diarrhea
00014	Bowel incontinence
00015	Risk for constipation
00016	Impaired urinary elimination
00017	Stress urinary incontinence
00018	Reflex urinary incontinence
00019	Urge urinary incontinence
00020	Functional urinary incontinence
00021	Total urinary incontinence
00022	Risk for urge urinary incontinence
00023	Urinary retention
00024	Ineffective tissue perfusion (specify type: renal, cerebral, cardiopulmonary, gastrointestinal, peripheral)

Taxonomy II code	Nursing diagnosis
00025	Risk for imbalanced fluid volume
00026	Excess fluid volume
00027	Deficient fluid volume
00028	Risk for deficient fluid volume
00029	Decreased cardiac output
00030	Impaired gas exchange
00031	Ineffective airway clearance
00032	Ineffective breathing pattern
00033	Impaired spontaneous ventilation
00034	Dysfunctional ventilatory weaning response
00035	Risk for injury
00036	Risk for suffocation
00037	Risk for poisoning
00038	Risk for trauma
00039	Risk for aspiration
00040	Risk for disuse syndrome
00041	Latex allergy response
00042	Risk for latex allergy response
00043	Ineffective protection
00044	Impaired tissue integrity
00045	Impaired oral mucous membrane
00046	Impaired skin integrity
00047	Risk for impaired skin integrity
00048	Impaired dentition
00049	Decreased intracranial adaptive capacity
00050	Disturbed energy field
00051	Impaired verbal communication
00052	Impaired social interaction
00053	Social isolation
00054	Risk for loneliness
00055	Ineffective role performance
00056	Impaired parenting
00057	Risk for impaired parenting
00058	Risk for impaired parent/infant/child attachment
00059	Sexual dysfunction
00060	Interrupted family processes
00061	Caregiver role strain
00062	Risk for caregiver role strain
00063	Dysfunctional family processes: Alcoholism
00064	Parental role conflict
00065	Ineffective sexuality patterns
00066	Spiritual distress
00067	Risk for spiritual distress
00068	Readiness for enhanced spiritual well-being
00069	Ineffective coping

Taxonomy II code	Nursing diagnosis
00070	Impaired adjustment
00071	Defensive coping
00072	Ineffective denial
00073	Disabled family coping
00074	Compromised family coping
00075	Readiness for enhanced family coping
00076	Readiness for enhanced community coping
00077	Ineffective community coping
00078	Ineffective therapeutic regimen management
00079	Noncompliance (specify)
00080	Ineffective family therapeutic regimen management
00081	Ineffective community therapeutic regimen management
00082	Effective therapeutic regimen management
00083	Decisional conflict (specify)
00084	Health-seeking behaviors (specify)
00085	Impaired physical mobility
00086	Risk for peripheral neurovascular dysfunction
00087	Risk for perioperative-positioning injury
00088	Impaired walking
00089	Impaired wheelchair mobility
00090	Impaired transfer ability
00091	Impaired bed mobility
00092	Activity intolerance
00093	Fatigue
00094	Risk for activity intolerance
00095	Disturbed sleep pattern
00096	Sleep deprivation
00097	Deficient diversional activity
00098	Impaired home maintenance
00099	Ineffective health maintenance
00100	Delayed surgical recovery
00101	Adult failure to thrive
00102	Feeding self-care deficit
00103	Impaired swallowing
00104	Ineffective breast-feeding
00105	Interrupted breast-feeding
00106	Effective breast-feeding
00107	Ineffective infant feeding pattern
00108	Bathing or hygiene self-care deficit
00109	Dressing or grooming self-care deficit
00110	Toileting self-care deficit
00111	Delayed growth and development
00112	Risk for delayed development
00113	Risk for disproportionate growth
00114	Relocation stress syndrome

Taxonomy II code	Nursing diagnosis
00115	Risk for disorganized infant behavior
00116	Disorganized infant behavior
00117	Readiness for enhanced organized infant behavior
00118	Disturbed body image
00119	Chronic low self-esteem
00120	Situational low self-esteem
00121	Disturbed personal identity
00122	Disturbed sensory perception (specify: visual, auditory, kinesthetic, gustatory, tactile, olfactory)
00123	Unilateral neglect
00124	Hopelessness
00125	Powerlessness
00126	Deficient knowledge (specify)
00127	Impaired environmental interpretation syndrome
00128	Acute confusion
00129	Chronic confusion
00130	Disturbed thought processes
00131	Impaired memory
00132	Acute pain
00133	Chronic pain
00134	Nausea
00135	Dysfunctional grieving
00136	Anticipatory grieving
00137	Chronic sorrow
00138	Risk for other-directed violence
00139	Risk for self-mutilation
00140	Risk for self-directed violence
00141	Posttrauma syndrome
00142	Rape-trauma syndrome
00143	Rape-trauma syndrome: Compound reaction
00144	Rape-trauma syndrome: Silent reaction
00145	Risk for posttrauma syndrome
00146	Anxiety
00147	Death anxiety
00148	Fear
00149	Risk for relocation stress syndrome
00150	Risk for suicide
00151	Self-mutilation
00152	Risk for powerlessness
00153	Risk for situational low self-esteem
00154	Wandering
00155	Risk for falls

Posttest

This posttest has been designed to evaluate your readiness to take the certification examination for psychiatric and mental health nursing. Similar in form and content to the actual examination, the posttest consists of 60 questions based on brief clinical situations; the questions will help sharpen your test-taking skills while assessing your knowledge of psychiatric and mental health nursing theory and practice.

You'll have 60 minutes to complete the posttest. To improve your chances of performing well, consider these suggestions:

● Read each clinical situation and question attentively; weigh the four options carefully; then select the option that best answers the question. (*Note:* In this posttest, options are lettered A, B, C, and D to aid in later identification of the correct answers and rationales. These letters don't appear in the certification examination.)

● If you have no idea of the correct answer, make an educated guess. (Only correct answers are counted in scoring the certification examination, so guessing is preferable to leaving a question unanswered.)

After you have completed the posttest or the 60-minute time limit expires, check your responses against the correct answers and rationales provided on pages 255 to 263.

Now, select a quiet room where you'll be undisturbed, set a timer for 60 minutes, and begin.

Questions

1. A nurse enters the dayroom and observes a rather buxom patient sitting at a table, playing cards with two male patients. The patient is wearing designer boots, a calf-length skirt, and a colorful vest over her otherwise bare chest. What's the nurse's *best* response to this patient?

○ **A.** "You need to go to your room and finish dressing."
○ **B.** "It isn't proper for you to be wearing only a vest."
○ **C.** "Where are your blouse, slip, and bra?"
○ **D.** "I'd like to see you for a few minutes in your room."

2. Your 35-year-old patient says that he never disagrees with anyone and that he has loved everyone he's ever known. What would be your *best* response to this patient?

○ **A.** "How do you manage to do that?"
○ **B.** "That's hard to believe. Most people couldn't do that."
○ **C.** "What do you do with feelings of anger or dissatisfaction?"
○ **D.** "How did you come to adopt such a way of life?"

3. Your 40-year-old patient, who's about to be discharged, says, "I'll bet you hated to graduate." What would be your *best* response to this patient?

○ **A.** "What prompts you to say that?"
○ **B.** "I really enjoyed my graduation."
○ **C.** "I hated saying good-bye to some of my friends."
○ **D.** "Tell me about how you felt when you graduated."

4. A male patient tried to run away from the hospital 2 days ago. As a result, his grounds privileges were revoked for 1 week. Today, he asks you to let him go for a short walk on the grounds. What would be your *best* response to the patient's request?

○ **A.** "Although I think it would be good for you to take a walk, your physician has taken away your grounds privileges."
○ **B.** "I understand your grounds privileges have been revoked. I'd be glad to do something with you on the unit."
○ **C.** "You decided to leave the hospital 2 days ago without permission. We can't allow you to go outside."
○ **D.** "You aren't allowed outside. It will be at least 5 more days before grounds privileges are restored."

5. You are sitting in the dayroom when a female patient begins to take off her clothing. What is the most reasonable inference for you to make?

○ **A.** She's hallucinating.
○ **B.** She's sexually preoccupied.
○ **C.** Her anxiety is at the severe or panic level.
○ **D.** The external environment is too stimulating.

6. The female patient described above continues to disrobe in the dayroom. Which of the following nursing actions would be the most therapeutic for such a patient?

○ **A.** Assist the patient in redressing; then take her to her room.
○ **B.** Ask the patient why she's disrobing in a public place.
○ **C.** Continue to observe the patient's behavior.
○ **D.** Clear the dayroom to give the patient privacy.

7. You're working with a patient who has just stimulated your anger by using a condescending tone of voice with you. Which of the following responses would be the most therapeutic way to acknowledge the effect on you?
- ○ **A.** "I feel angry when I hear that tone of voice."
- ○ **B.** "You make me so angry when you talk to me that way."
- ○ **C.** "Are you trying to make me angry?"
- ○ **D.** "Why do you do that with me?"

8. A 36-year-old male patient has just spent the past 10 minutes complaining about the hospital and his physician; he concludes his monologue by saying, "The nurses around here are insensitive and incompetent." What's your *best* response to the patient?
- ○ **A.** "It's difficult to be sensitive to a person who complains as you do."
- ○ **B.** "I don't appreciate your verbal abusiveness. We'll talk later when you cool down."
- ○ **C.** "Sometimes the things we can't tolerate in others are the very things we can't tolerate in ourselves."
- ○ **D.** "Give me a specific example of a nurse being insensitive or incompetent."

9. A patient on your unit says that the Mafia has a "contract" out on him. He refuses to leave his semiprivate room and insists on frisking his roommate before allowing him to enter. Which of the following actions should you take *first*?
- ○ **A.** Have the patient transferred to a private room.
- ○ **B.** Acknowledge the patient's fear when he refuses to leave his room or wants to frisk his roommate.
- ○ **C.** Transfer the roommate to another room.
- ○ **D.** Lock the patient out of his room for a short time each day so that he can see that he's safe.

10. You're working with a young woman who has acute schizophrenia. As you approach her, you notice that she's sitting on her bed in a puddle of urine. She's playing in it, smiling, and softly singing a children's song. Which of the following nursing actions would be the *best* one to take?
- ○ **A.** Admonish her for not using the bathroom.
- ○ **B.** Firmly tell her that her behavior is unacceptable.
- ○ **C.** Ask her if she's ready to get cleaned up now.
- ○ **D.** Help her to the shower, and change the bedclothes.

11. A 38-year-old female patient has been hospitalized twice previously for episodes of hypomania (bipolar disorder). She talks incessantly in an exhilarated manner and jumps from one activity to another, showing a limited concentration span. She also intrudes on the activities of others. At one point, the woman approaches an immobilized, depressed patient and enthusiastically invites him to dance. What's the nurse's *best* intervention?

○ **A.** Tell the patient that her behavior is inappropriate.
○ **B.** Ask the other patient how he feels about dancing with the female patient.
○ **C.** Do nothing if the other patient appears comfortable.
○ **D.** Take the patient to a quiet environment, and engage her in a structured activity.

12. One of your patients is suffering from depression. He refuses to go to occupational therapy (OT) because he says it's boring. Which of the following actions would be the *best* one for you to take?

○ **A.** State firmly that you will escort him to OT.
○ **B.** Arrange with OT for the patient to do a project on the unit.
○ **C.** Ask the patient to talk about why OT is boring.
○ **D.** Arrange for the patient not to attend OT until he feels better.

13. A female patient with depression says that she's "no good" and tells you to "spend your time with someone else." Which of the following responses would be the most therapeutic for this patient?

○ **A.** "I'm going to stay with you for the next 15 minutes."
○ **B.** "Because I'm assigned to you, I'll stay with you."
○ **C.** "Why do you put yourself down like that?"
○ **D.** "What do you mean when you say that you're no good?"

14. A 42-year-old male patient returns to the hospital at 9 p.m. from a city day pass. He's 3 hours late. The nurse smells alcohol on his breath. His speech is slurred, and his gait is unsteady. What would be the nurse's *best* response to this patient?

○ **A.** "Why are you 3 hours late in returning from your city day pass?"
○ **B.** "How much did you drink tonight? You know drinking is against the rules."
○ **C.** "I'm disappointed that you haven't been more responsible with your city day pass."
○ **D.** "I want you to go to bed now. We'll talk in the morning."

15. A patient on your unit tells you that his wife's nagging really gets on his nerves. He asks if you will talk with her about her nagging during their family session tomorrow afternoon. Which of the following responses would be the most therapeutic to the patient?

- ○ **A.** "Tell me more specifically about her complaints."
- ○ **B.** "Can you think why she might nag you so much?"
- ○ **C.** "I'll help you think about how to bring this up yourself tomorrow afternoon."
- ○ **D.** "Why do you want me to initiate this in tomorrow's session rather than you?"

16. One of your new patients is experiencing delusions. Which of the following nursing actions is important when working with a delusional patient?

- ○ **A.** Question the patient about the delusion.
- ○ **B.** Point out to the patient why the delusion is false.
- ○ **C.** Go along with the delusion until the patient's anxiety decreases.
- ○ **D.** Refocus the patient toward a structured activity.

17. A 32-year-old woman is admitted to the psychiatric unit after experiencing a conversion reaction. The nurse initially establishes short- and long-term goals. Which of the following statements is a long-term goal?

- ○ **A.** The patient will verbalize her feelings and anxiety.
- ○ **B.** The patient will participate in unit activities.
- ○ **C.** The patient will gain insight into her paralysis.
- ○ **D.** The patient will perform self-care.

18. During the working phase of the nurse-patient relationship, the patient says to her primary nurse, "You think I could walk if I wanted to, don't you?" What would be the nurse's *best* response?

- ○ **A.** "Yes, if you really wanted to, you could."
- ○ **B.** "Tell me why you're concerned about what I think."
- ○ **C.** "Do you think you could walk if you wanted to?"
- ○ **D.** "I think you're unable to walk now, whatever the cause."

19. Because of an illness in your extended family, you missed your last appointment with a patient on a psychiatric unit. As you enter the unit today, the patient rushes toward you and says in a loud and pressured tone of voice, "I can't help you." Which of the following responses would be the *best* one to make?

- ○ **A.** "Who told you why I wasn't here last time?"
- ○ **B.** "How do you feel about my missing our last meeting?"
- ○ **C.** "I'm not sure what you mean when you say you can't help me."
- ○ **D.** "Thank you for your concern about my being absent."

20. A young female patient who's in a psychiatric facility stiffly walks up to the nurse and says in a flat tone of voice, "I'm dead. The staff just killed me." Which of the following responses would be the *most* therapeutic?

○ **A.** "What did the staff do to kill you?"

○ **B.** "You look like you're alive to me."

○ **C.** "Would you like to lie down for a while?"

○ **D.** "I'm not sure what you mean."

21. A patient reports to her therapy group that she has begun to practice a conscious relaxation technique. She's pleased with its effectiveness in reducing her need to wash her hands. One member responds by saying that conscious relaxation is a bunch of nonsense. A nurse is serving as group leader. Which of the following interventions would be the *best* one for the nurse to make at this point?

○ **A.** Smile and change the focus of discussion.

○ **B.** Ask the group member why he thinks the technique worked so well for the patient.

○ **C.** Foster group cohesiveness by asking the member to keep negative opinions to himself.

○ **D.** Ask the member to share his understanding of and experience with conscious relaxation.

22. A patient on the psychiatric unit has obtained a Sunday pass to go to a family reunion picnic. He's taking fluphenazine (Prolixin). The nurse gives the patient instructions to follow while at the picnic. Which of the following statements by the patient shows an understanding of the teaching?

○ **A.** "I'll wear plenty of sunscreen at the picnic."

○ **B.** "I'll drink an extra quart of fluid at the picnic."

○ **C.** "I'll avoid eating cheese at the picnic."

○ **D.** "I'll engage in picnic activities only in a limited manner."

23. A 47-year-old man is suffering from acute exogenous depression that developed after his wife's death. He's taking phenelzine sulfate (Nardil), a monoamine oxidase (MAO) inhibitor, to control symptoms of the depression. Other than his current problem, he has no history of mental or physical illness. He has been admitted to the hospital with a marked blood pressure elevation. Your initial assessment would include a thorough neurologic evaluation. What's the rationale for such an evaluation?

○ **A.** Acute exogenous depression is characterized by enhanced platelet activity and cerebrovascular accidents.

○ **B.** Acute exogenous depression, when treated with an MAO inhibitor, can result in permanent neurologic impairment if therapeutic dosages are exceeded.

○ **C.** MAO inhibitors are associated with acute hypertensive crisis related to the intake of certain foods and drugs.

○ **D.** Blood pressure elevation may signal the onset of the depression's manic phase.

24. A patient has been on your nursing unit for 1 week. Her nighttime confusion and wandering have decreased but continue to occur at least once each night. During a team meeting, a staff member recommends that the patient be placed in restraints at night. What would be your *best* response?

- ○ **A.** "Restraints are used only to protect the health and safety of patients."
- ○ **B.** "Restraints may be used for purposes of discipline."
- ○ **C.** "Restraints may be used to control a patient's verbal outbursts."
- ○ **D.** "Restraints are effective in reducing the number of patient falls."

25. A patient, age 19, just arrived on your psychiatric unit from the emergency department. Unemployed, he has been living at home with his parents. His diagnosis is personality disorder, and he exhibits manipulative behavior. You go over the unit rules with him. The patient asks, "Can I go to the snack shop just one time, and then I'll answer whatever questions you have?" What would be your *best* response to this patient?

- ○ **A.** "Okay, but hurry up. I need to finish your assessment."
- ○ **B.** "Okay, but only for 5 minutes."
- ○ **C.** "No, you can't go."
- ○ **D.** "No, you can't go. The rules here are for everyone."

26. A 22-year-old female patient has been diagnosed with antisocial personality disorder. She has been having problems since age 15, when she ran away from home. The patient has had two broken marriages and can't keep a job for more than 2 months. She has had difficulties with the law because of drug abuse and writing bad checks. She has just broken another unit rule, and her phone privileges have been revoked. The patient asks the nurse, "Can't I just make one more phone call?" What would be the nurse's *best* response?

- ○ **A.** "Okay, but don't talk too long."
- ○ **B.** "Okay, if you promise to obey the rules for the rest of the day."
- ○ **C.** "No, you can't. The rules apply equally to everyone, and you broke them."
- ○ **D.** "No, you can't. Go watch television."

27. At the start of a group therapy session, a patient tells you that another patient has been discussing group business with people who aren't in the group. The patient says she's no longer willing to share anything in the group because of the other patient's "big mouth." What would be your *best* response to this patient?

- ○ **A.** "I want you to tell the person who did this what you've just told me."
- ○ **B.** "How do you know that this person has discussed group business with others?"
- ○ **C.** "I would also be hesitant about sharing anything else in the group."
- ○ **D.** "How do you feel about what this person did?"

28. An 8-year-old girl hasn't gone to school for 3 weeks. Each morning she says she feels sick and has refused to get out of bed. The girl's mother brings her to the mental health clinic. Which of the following actions is *most* important during your first interview with the girl's mother?

- ○ **A.** Reassure her that this is probably a phase that her daughter will soon pass through.
- ○ **B.** Ask her to identify tensions in the home that could be precipitating the daughter's behavior.
- ○ **C.** Ask her to describe any changes that occurred before the daughter's symptoms developed.
- ○ **D.** Have her describe each family member's relationship with the daughter.

29. What action would be appropriate during your first interview with the daughter?

- ○ **A.** Ask her why she doesn't like school anymore.
- ○ **B.** Have her describe how things were for her immediately before she started not wanting to go to school anymore.
- ○ **C.** Tell her that it's okay for her to be afraid to go to school but that she will have to start going back.
- ○ **D.** Reassure her that even though things may not be right in her life just now, they soon will be.

30. A nurse is the leader of an inpatient therapy group. One group member accuses the nurse of being far too pushy and says that the nurse doesn't have the right to pressure anyone in the group. Which of the following responses would be *most* likely to help the patient remain nondefensive?

- ○ **A.** "I'm sensing that you're uncomfortable in the group."
- ○ **B.** "Why are you feeling pressured and pushed by me?"
- ○ **C.** "Can you tell me exactly what it is that's bothering you?"
- ○ **D.** "Tell me about one time when you felt pushed or pressured."

31. You're working on an eating disorder hot line. A 27-year-old woman calls in, crying; she says that she feels miserable about her disgusting habit of binging and vomiting. She asks if you can help her. What would be your *best* response?

- ○ **A.** "You did the right thing by calling the hot line. We can help you."
- ○ **B.** "Tell me about your binging and vomiting. Talking about it will help you."
- ○ **C.** "Let me give you the name and number of a good therapist. Will you call him?"
- ○ **D.** "I'm a nurse, and I want you to come to our clinic immediately. I'll be waiting for you."

32. A female patient, age 59, has been diagnosed with Alzheimer's disease. She has been wearing the same dirty and torn undergarments for several days. The nurse contacts her daughters and asks them to bring in other clothing. Which of the following interventions would *best* prevent further regression in the patient's personal hygiene habits?
- ○ **A.** Encourage the patient to perform as much self-care as she can.
- ○ **B.** Make the patient assume responsibility for her physical care.
- ○ **C.** Assign a staff member to take over the patient's physical care.
- ○ **D.** Accept the patient's need to go without bathing and to wear dirty clothing if she so desires.

33. A patient with Alzheimer's disease becomes verbally and physically abusive when the nurse enters her room to assist with her daily care. Which of the following interventions should the nurse engage in *first*?
- ○ **A.** Check orders for physical and chemical restraints.
- ○ **B.** Set firm limits verbally.
- ○ **C.** Give clear directions while gently securing the patient's arms to prevent her from hitting the nurse.
- ○ **D.** Leave the room and let the angry, hostile behavior work itself out.

34. A 28-year-old accountant is admitted to the neurologic unit after a sudden onset of blindness the day before an important project is due for her boss. Preliminary evaluation and testing reveal no positive findings. The physician's initial reaction is that the patient may be demonstrating a defense mechanism. Which of the following defense mechanisms might the patient be using?
- ○ **A.** Repression
- ○ **B.** Transference
- ○ **C.** Reaction formation
- ○ **D.** Conversion

35. A woman, age 40, is brought to the hospital by her husband because she has refused to get out of bed for 2 days. She won't eat, has been neglecting her household responsibilities, and is tired all the time. Her diagnosis on admission is major depression. The woman is being interviewed by the admitting nurse. Which of the following questions would be *most* appropriate for the nurse to ask at this time?
- ○ **A.** "What has been troubling you?"
- ○ **B.** "Why do you dislike yourself?"
- ○ **C.** "How do you feel about your life?"
- ○ **D.** "What can we do to help?"

36. A patient diagnosed with major depression begins to improve and participates in treatment programs on the unit. You recognize that the patient is ready for discharge when she:
- ○ **A.** asks the staff for advice about how to handle her future.
- ○ **B.** speaks to her employer about returning to work.
- ○ **C.** identifies her weaknesses and plans to work on them.
- ○ **D.** discusses her plan to return home and continue outpatient treatment.

37. An abused child is expected to stay on your unit for 3 to 4 weeks. Which of the following nursing assignments would be *best* for this patient?
- ○ **A.** A different primary nurse each day
- ○ **B.** A primary nurse who's transferring next week to another unit
- ○ **C.** The same primary nurse each day
- ○ **D.** A new primary nurse every 3 days

38. A 24-year-old secretary is transferred to your psychiatric unit. Her husband says that she has been overeating and that she vomits soon after she eats. Her weight stays about the same. Which of the following medical diagnoses would apply in this case?
- ○ **A.** Anorexia nervosa
- ○ **B.** Bulimia
- ○ **C.** Bulimarexia
- ○ **D.** Dysthymia

39. A 45-year-old housewife has been treated for major depression for the past 15 years. She reports to her physician that she has been experiencing complications from her current antidepressant, so the physician prescribes an MAO inhibitor instead. Which of the following foods should the patient be instructed to avoid once she begins taking the MAO inhibitor?
- ○ **A.** Smoked salmon
- ○ **B.** Milk and egg products
- ○ **C.** Honey
- ○ **D.** Dried nuts

40. After teaching a patient about the adverse effects associated with certain foods and MAO inhibitors, you begin to caution her about possible interactions between MAOs and other drugs. Which of the following drugs should the patient avoid while taking an MAO inhibitor?
- ○ **A.** Aspirin
- ○ **B.** Anticoagulants
- ○ **C.** Antihistamines
- ○ **D.** Antihypertensives

41. A woman, age 72, frequently wanders away from home and is unable to provide directions on how to return. What is the *best* instruction to the woman's daughter on how to ensure her safety?
- ○ **A.** "Your mother's condition is temporary; it will soon pass."
- ○ **B.** "If I were you, I'd move in with your mother."
- ○ **C.** "It's best that you have your mother committed."
- ○ **D.** "It's important that someone is available at all times for your mother's safety."

42. A 15-year-old girl was admitted to the eating disorders unit 2 days ago. She's 5'6" (1.7 m) tall and weighs 92 lb (41.7 kg). You're the girl's primary nurse and will be having your first one-on-one session with her today. What represents the *most* important information that you should gather from the girl during this first session?

○ **A.** A detailed history of her eating habits
○ **B.** How she views her current situation
○ **C.** What she expects to achieve during hospitalization
○ **D.** How she views herself in relation to her peers

43. Since being admitted to the eating disorders unit, a 15-year-old female patient has dropped from 92 lb to 89 lb (40.4 kg). Which of the following nursing actions would be *best* at this point?

○ **A.** Place the patient on a behavior modification program.
○ **B.** Place the patient on bed rest until she regains the 3 lb (1.4 kg).
○ **C.** Tell the patient that you're concerned about the 3-lb loss.
○ **D.** Ask the patient which foods she would feel most comfortable eating.

44. After 4 weeks, the patient's weight increases from 89 lb to 93 lb (42.2 kg). Which of the following nursing actions would be the *best* one to take now?

○ **A.** Suggest that the patient be discharged and treated on an outpatient basis.
○ **B.** Set weekly treatment goals for the patient to review in group therapy.
○ **C.** Negotiate with the patient about the continuing terms of the treatment plan.
○ **D.** Engage in weekly psychotherapy sessions with the patient and her family.

45. A very shy, retiring patient hands you several capsules he found "on the floor." Several patients are receiving this particular medication. Which of the following actions should you take *first*?

○ **A.** Restrict all patient privileges until you find out what's happening.
○ **B.** Initiate a unit-wide search to determine whether more drugs can be found.
○ **C.** Observe all patients carefully during and after they receive the medication in question.
○ **D.** Call all the patients together, and ask if anyone knows how these capsules got on the floor.

46. One of your patients tells you that nothing good has ever happened to her. You use a cognitive approach in your work with patients. Which of the following responses represents the cognitive approach?

○ **A.** "You must feel terrible."
○ **B.** "How have you come to that conclusion?"
○ **C.** "Hasn't your relationship with me been good?"
○ **D.** "How does that make you feel?"

47. A patient asks you if it's okay for him to leave your one-on-one session to get a drink of water. One of the patient's treatment goals is to promote personal growth. What would be the *best* response to the patient's question?

○ **A.** "Whether or not you get a drink is your decision."
○ **B.** "Your leaving to get a drink would be disruptive."
○ **C.** "We're almost finished; do you think you can wait?"
○ **D.** "You should have taken care of that before we started."

48. Your patient's mother died unexpectedly about 8 months ago. The patient still has many regrets about not coming to closure with her mother over two specific issues. You plan to use a Gestalt approach when working with the patient. Which of the following interventions represents the Gestalt approach?

○ **A.** Change the ego state from which the patient operates.
○ **B.** Teach the patient about the stages of grieving.
○ **C.** Identify the thoughts leading to the patient's distress.
○ **D.** Have the patient "talk" to her mother.

49. A 24-year-old man is an intrusive patient, constantly invading the physical and social spaces of staff and peers. He doesn't comprehend that his behavior is inappropriate. Which of the following descriptions represents the Sullivanian theory?

○ **A.** The patient experiences severe-level anxiety.
○ **B.** The patient operates in the prototaxic mode.
○ **C.** The patient exhibits problems with intimacy versus isolation.
○ **D.** The patient has an ineffective ego and overactive id.

50. A patient is admitted to the oncology unit for treatment of uterine cancer. Routine laboratory tests reveal a total white blood cell count below normal limits, with a marked reduction in the neutrophil count. Her physician orders lithium carbonate, 300 mg three times a day (t.i.d.) by mouth. When the drug is administered for the first time, her husband becomes angry and follows you out into the hallway. He whispers loudly, "That drug is for crazy people. My wife has cancer!" What is your *best* response to the patient's husband?

○ **A.** "We understand your wife has cancer. This drug is being given for other purposes."
○ **B.** "Calm down. Would you like to talk about it?"
○ **C.** "You're angry because you think we don't know what's wrong with your wife."
○ **D.** "I'm sorry you're upset. Let me explain why the physician ordered lithium."

51. The patient has been receiving lithium for 2 weeks. She has also been receiving a number of chemotherapeutic drugs that cause her to feel nauseated and anorexic, making it difficult to distinguish the early signs of lithium toxicity. Which of the following signs would indicate lithium toxicity at serum drug levels below 1.5 mEq/L?

- ○ **A.** Hyperpyrexia
- ○ **B.** Marked analgesia and lethargy
- ○ **C.** Hypotonic reflexes with muscle weakness
- ○ **D.** Renal failure

52. A patient on an inpatient psychiatric unit at a community mental health center has a history of aggression. One of the nurses observes the patient continually pacing up and down the hallway. What would be the nurse's *best* response?

- ○ **A.** "If you can't relax, you could go to your room."
- ○ **B.** "Would you like your antianxiety medication now?"
- ○ **C.** "You're pacing. What's going on?"
- ○ **D.** "Let's go play a game of pool."

53. A patient who was voluntarily admitted asks to be discharged from the hospital against medical advice. What *must* the nurse assess before the patient is discharged?

- ○ **A.** Ability to self-care
- ○ **B.** Danger to self and others
- ○ **C.** Level of psychosis
- ○ **D.** Intended compliance with treatment after discharge

54. A 24-year-old schizophrenic patient is admitted to the unit in a catatonic state. The physician prescribes haloperidol (Haldol), 5 mg t.i.d. Four days after admission, the patient comes out of the coma and gradually begins to take care of herself. She says that the FBI is after her because she was a key figure in a political scandal involving the President of the United States. What would be the nurse's *best* response?

- ○ **A.** "How long have you known the President?"
- ○ **B.** "You don't know the President."
- ○ **C.** "Why do you think the FBI would be looking for you here?"
- ○ **D.** "You must feel important. May I accompany you to breakfast?"

55. A 45-year-old accountant has been admitted to the hospital because of extreme agitation. He thinks that he must pace the floor a specific number of times each day or "something terrible" will happen to him. He has engaged in this behavior most of his adult life. What would be the *most* appropriate response for the nurse to make?

- ○ **A.** "Nothing will happen to you. You must stop this behavior."
- ○ **B.** "Are you looking for attention? There are other ways you can get this attention."
- ○ **C.** "This behavior has created some difficulty for you. It might help if we talked about why you find it necessary to do this."
- ○ **D.** "I understand your need to work off excess energy."

56. A 39-year-old man is suffering from depression. He says, "I'm a failure. I can't even cope with little things anymore." Which of the following statements would be the *most* appropriate nursing response?

- ○ **A.** "Do you feel like you don't deserve to feel good about yourself?"
- ○ **B.** "I know you feel like that now, but you'll feel differently when you get better."
- ○ **C.** "What has happened to make you feel like such a failure?"
- ○ **D.** "It sounds as if you're feeling pretty overwhelmed right now."

57. A woman comes into the emergency services department of the community mental health center. Pleadingly she says to the nurse, "Make my husband stop drinking." What would be the nurse's *best* response?

- ○ **A.** "Tell me exactly why you're so concerned about your husband's drinking."
- ○ **B.** "I can't do anything about your husband's drinking unless he comes here for help."
- ○ **C.** "I can see you're feeling distraught. Tell me exactly what made you come here today."
- ○ **D.** "I can see you're feeling distraught. It's hard to live with someone who abuses alcohol."

58. You've been working with a patient who has an anxiety disorder. During one of your meetings, the patient abruptly says, "I really love you." What would be your *best* response?

- ○ **A.** "Why do you think you love me?"
- ○ **B.** "What do you mean you love me? Are you sure?"
- ○ **C.** "I can sense you have strong feelings about me. Let's talk about that."
- ○ **D.** "It's nice to share feelings with others. What other feelings could we share?"

59. A 15-year-old patient with anorexia nervosa asks you if she has done any permanent damage to her body. Which of the following responses would be the *most* therapeutic reply?

- ○ **A.** "It's too early to determine that yet."
- ○ **B.** "Have you asked your physician that question?"
- ○ **C.** "What has prompted you to ask that question?"
- ○ **D.** "Did someone say you've damaged your body?"

60. An acutely manic patient kisses you on the mouth and asks you to marry him. You're taken by surprise. How should you respond?

- ○ **A.** Seclude him for his inappropriate behavior.
- ○ **B.** Ask him what he's trying to prove by his behavior.
- ○ **C.** Have him help you fold some laundry.
- ○ **D.** Tell him that you find his behavior offensive.

Answers and rationales

The question number appears in boldface type, followed by the correct answer. The text then provides rationales for correct answers and, where appropriate, for incorrect options.

1. Correct answer: D Requesting a private conversation demonstrates respect for the patient while removing her from an embarrassing situation. Option A is incorrect because the patient would have worn more clothing if she thought that she needed it; because her anxiety level is severe, she can't independently follow through with instructions. Options B and C are incorrect because they are insensitive to the social context in which the patient's behavior is occurring.

2. Correct answer: D Inquiring about the patient's way of life allows for further exploration of the message he's trying to convey. Option A has too narrow a focus and doesn't permit maximal exploration of the patient's experience. Option B is incorrect because the patient could misinterpret it as a challenge and become more defensive than he already is. Option C is incorrect because the nurse shouldn't identify the patient's feelings for him.

3. Correct answer: A Asking the patient to reveal what prompted his remark allows for further exploration of his statement. Options B and C serve as blocks to such exploration, improperly focusing on the nurse's feelings rather than the patient's. Option D is too concrete a response and misses the point.

4. Correct answer: B This response restates the imposed limitation without demeaning the patient and conveys the nurse's willingness to spend time with the patient. Option A is incorrect because the nurse, in assigning sole responsibility for the revocation to the physician, would be engaging in staff splitting. Option C implies that the staff is unable to make decisions; the use of the word "can't" implies helplessness. Although Option D adequately restates the imposed limitation, it gives no indication of the nurse's willingness to spend time with the patient.

5. Correct answer: C Patients with mild or moderate anxiety don't behave in socially inappropriate ways, so this patient's anxiety must be at the severe or panic level. Options A, B, and D are all incorrect because the clinical situation doesn't include sufficient data to support these inferences.

6. Correct answer: A The most therapeutic nursing action would be to help the patient get dressed and then take her to her room. The nurse shouldn't permit the patient to do anything in public that will embarrass the patient later. Option B is incorrect because the patient's anxiety level doesn't permit her to solve problems independently. Option C is incorrect because the patient's anxiety is high enough that she'll continue her behavior and further embarrass herself. Option D doesn't set appropriate limits on her socially inappropriate behavior.

7. **Correct answer: A** This response (known as an "I" message, as opposed to a "you" message) allows you to provide feedback without making the patient responsible for your reaction. Option B is accusatory and blocks communication. Option C is a challenging remark that can lead to power struggles, lower the patient's self-esteem, and block opportunities for open communication. Option D is incorrect because "why" questions put the patient on the defensive.

8. **Correct answer: D** Asking the patient to support his contention with a concrete example compels him to specify events and may enhance his ability to view the situation more objectively. Option A may only serve to exacerbate the patient's already negative behavior. Option B halts the conversation, blocking therapeutic communication. Option C is too confrontational.

9. **Correct answer: B** Acknowledging underlying feelings may help defuse the patient's anxiety without promoting his delusional thinking. This, in turn, may help the patient distinguish between his emotional state and external reality. Options A and C aren't the preferred actions because transferring either patient to another room would validate the patient's delusional thinking. (If Option B doesn't work, however, then Option C would be the next best action, to protect the roommate and to control the patient's anxiety.) Option D—locking the patient out of his room—would probably further escalate his anxiety and stimulate aggressive acting-out behavior; it also would deprive him of a place where he could feel safe.

10. **Correct answer: D** The patient has panic-level anxiety. You must help her meet self-care needs. Options A, B, and C are inappropriate for a patient with panic anxiety; she couldn't "hear" you, and she would require more structure and assistance than those options afford.

11. **Correct answer: D** Because the patient can't set limits on her own behavior, the nurse must do so. Structured activities tend to benefit patients with bipolar disorder, who typically need assistance in appropriately channeling their energy. Option A insufficiently addresses the patient's severe anxiety level. Option B not only puts the other patient in an awkward position but also condones the inappropriate behavior. Option C fails to address the inappropriate behavior, which, if left unchecked, will eventually create anxiety in others who are in her immediate environment.

12. **Correct answer: A** If given the chance, a depressed patient typically elects to remain immobilized. You must insist that the patient participate in occupational therapy (OT). Option B validates and reinforces the patient's desire to avoid going to OT. Option C addresses an invalid issue (most things bore de-

pressed people) while avoiding the real issue (the patient's need for therapy). Option D incorrectly suggests that the patient isn't capable of participating in OT, further undermining an already lowered self-esteem.

13. Correct answer: A This response conveys your interest in the patient while firmly communicating that you won't be pushed away. Option B suggests that staying with the patient is a duty you're performing unwillingly, which may further diminish her already low self-esteem. Options C and D inappropriately focus on the negative by inviting the patient to expand on the reasons why she's no good, reinforcing her negative self-image.

14. Correct answer: D The patient can best process his behavior when he's no longer under the influence of alcohol. Option A is incorrect because the patient (who's intoxicated and may be experiencing a blackout) may invent excuses for his whereabouts. Option B is incorrect because any consumption of alcohol by the patient is unacceptable; the amount is irrelevant. Option C is inappropriate because the nurse's statement is judgmental.

15. Correct answer: C The patient needs to learn how to communicate directly with his wife about her behavior. Your assistance will enable him to practice a new skill and will communicate your confidence in his ability to confront this situation directly. Options A and B inappropriately direct attention away from the patient and toward his wife, who isn't present. Option D implies that there might be a legitimate reason for you to assume responsibility for something that rightfully belongs to the patient. Instead of focusing on his problems, he'll waste precious time convincing you why you should do his work.

16. Correct answer: D Refocusing the patient toward a structured activity reinforces reality. Options A and C are incorrect because the nurse shouldn't make delusions seem real. Option B is futile; the more the nurse tries to disprove the delusion, the more the patient will cling to it.

17. Correct answer: C Having the patient gain insight into her paralysis is the only long-term goal listed. Options A, B, and D are short-term goals.

18. Correct answer: D This response answers the question honestly and nonjudgmentally and helps to preserve the patient's self-esteem. Option A is an open and candid response but diminishes the patient's self-esteem. Option B doesn't answer the patient's question and isn't helpful. Option C would increase the patient's anxiety because her inability to walk is directly related to an unconscious psychological conflict that hasn't been resolved.

19. Correct answer: C This response seeks clarification about what the patient thinks she should be doing for the nurse; it also allows for exploration of possible feelings of helplessness or uselessness in past situations. Options A, B, and D don't address the patient's comment that she can't help the nurse. Option D also blocks further exploration of the patient's feelings.

20. Correct answer: D This response seeks further clarification of the patient's comment. Option A inappropriately validates the patient's misperception. Option B denies the patient's experience. Option C ignores the patient's statement.

21. Correct answer: D This response seeks first to clarify the group member's experience and then to provide an opportunity for the group leader or another member to explain the purpose of conscious relaxation. Option A ignores the issue being discussed. Option B takes the focus away from the patient's concern. Option C doesn't foster group cohesiveness; negative opinions are valid and shouldn't be suppressed.

22. Correct answer: A Fluphenazine, an antipsychotic drug, can cause photosensitivity and severe sunburn. Options B and C are incorrect because they don't influence the effects of antipsychotic drugs. Option D is incorrect because antipsychotic drugs don't affect one's ability to engage in usual picnic activities.

23. Correct answer: C In combination with monoamine oxidase (MAO) inhibitors, tyramine (a substance found in certain foods and drugs) can cause an acute hypertensive crisis. Option A is incorrect because MAO inhibitors have no effect on platelet activity. Option B is incorrect because MAO inhibitors affect the storage of neurohormones; they have no direct effect on nerve cells and no permanent effect on the body. Option D is incorrect because people with exogenous depression aren't prone to manic episodes.

24. Correct answer: A Existing laws stipulate the acceptable practices involved in the use of restraints. Protecting the health and safety of the patient is the primary reason to use restraints. Options B and C are incorrect because the laws expressly prohibit the use of restraints to control or discipline a patient. Option D is incorrect in light of recent research showing that restraints don't significantly reduce patient falls.

25. Correct answer: D This response sets appropriate limits. Options A and B give in to the patient's manipulative behavior. Option C doesn't provide an explanation for the refusal.

26. Correct answer: C This response enforces the unit rules and explains why the patient isn't permitted to use the phone. Options A and B don't encourage the patient to follow rules. Option D doesn't explain why the patient's request has been refused.

27. Correct answer: A This response forces the patient to validate her perception directly with other group members. Adult behavior includes learning how to be assertive without being hostile. Options B, C, and D don't assist the patient in learning this task.

28. Correct answer: C   This response allows you to assess what could have precipitated the girl's change in behavior. Option A is incorrect because it provides false reassurance. Option B is incorrect because it makes an assumption without gathering the necessary data. Option D would yield helpful information but not the most important information needed.

29. Correct answer: B   You need to assess what precipitated the daughter's anxious behavior. Option A is incorrect because the daughter may not be able to answer this question. Option C is an inappropriate comment to make in the initial interview. Option D offers the patient false reassurance.

30. Correct answer: D   This response compels the patient to provide a specific example, which may help the patient to view the situation more objectively. Option A may be too threatening to the patient. Option B could lead to denial if the patient feels directly threatened. Option C is inappropriate; if the patient knew what was bothering him, he would act differently.

31. Correct answer: D   This response conveys immediate interest and concern; it tells the caller that you're willing to get involved and provide tangible assistance. Option A doesn't prompt the caller to take action. Option B is incorrect because talking about the problem won't solve it. Option C is a brush-off, and the caller may hesitate to call someone else.

32. Correct answer: A   This response increases the patient's orientation and provides a safe environment while establishing a nurse-patient relationship based on trust. Patients with organic mental syndromes tend to fluctuate frequently in terms of their capabilities. Option B would be difficult to accomplish because of the patient's confusion. Options C and D diminish the patient's independence and self-esteem. Option D also ignores the patient's hygiene and grooming needs.

33. Correct answer: B   Clear limits protect the patient, staff, and others, and sometimes a verbally and physically abusive patient responds to verbal controls. Option A (using restraints to reduce anxiety and control behavior) would be considered only as a last resort, if at all. Option C invades the patient's personal space, which might escalate unacceptable behavior. Option D invites the possibility of injury if the patient strikes out at the nurse or an imagined threat.

34. Correct answer: D   When feelings become unbearable, the patient may rechannel them into physical symptoms. Conversion is a defense mechanism that usually appears shortly after a traumatic or conflict-producing event. The symptoms have no organic cause and often provide attention or an excuse. Repression (Option A) is a defense mechanism by which a person unconsciously keeps unwanted feelings from entering awareness. Transference (Option B) is a defense mechanism by which a person projects feelings, thoughts, and wishes onto others; it can be positive or negative. Reaction formation (Option C) is a defense mechanism by which a person alleviates unresolved emotional conflicts by reinforcing one feeling or impulse and repressing another, thereby disguising the true feelings from the self.

35. Correct answer: C   The nurse must develop nursing interventions based on the patient's perceived problems and feelings. Option A asks the patient to draw a conclusion, which may be difficult for her to do at this time. Option B asks a "why" question, which can place the patient in a defensive position. Option D requires the patient to find possible solutions, which is beyond the scope of her present abilities.

36. Correct answer: D   The patient's plan to return home and continue outpatient treatment indicates that she's willing to assume responsibility for her health. Option A implies an unwillingness to accept responsibility. Option B is a positive step, but it won't help the patient comprehensively. Option C involves short-term steps taken well before discharge.

37. Correct answer: C   Assigning the same primary nurse every day will provide continuity of care and facilitate the development of trust in the nurse-patient relationship. Options A, B, and D aren't in the best interest of the patient and won't promote a trusting relationship.

38. Correct answer: B   The patient exhibits binging and purging, common signs of bulimia. Option A is incorrect because the patient hasn't experienced weight loss, a common sign of anorexia nervosa. With bulimarexia (Option C), one would expect to see symptoms of both anorexia nervosa and bulimia. Dysthymia (Option D) is a type of depression.

39. Correct answer: A   Smoked salmon contains tyramine, a substance that can produce a hypertensive crisis if ingested in a large enough amount by a person taking an MAO inhibitor. The foods listed in the other options don't contain tyramine.

40. Correct answer: D   Hypotension is an adverse effect of MAO inhibitors. Combining an antihypertensive medication with an MAO inhibitor could lead to heart failure. Options A, B, and C wouldn't produce a drug-drug interaction.

41. Correct answer: D   This response specifies the conditions necessary for the woman to be safe while allowing the daughter to determine how she wants to implement the plan. Option A gives false information. Options B and C impose personal values on the patient's daughter.

42. Correct answer: B   The patient's view of her situation determines her behaviors. The nurse can't plan effective care without first understanding this viewpoint. Option A incorrectly focuses on food and eating habits, which aren't the real issue; the patient's underlying feelings actually precipitated the eating disorder. Option C is premature. The patient doesn't know what she expects to achieve during hospitalization. She's probably anxious about being "forced" to gain weight and may try to "play games" with the nurse. Option D is also premature. The first session between the patient and the nurse should be devoted to establishing rapport and defining the nature of their relationship.

43. Correct answer: B Bed rest will conserve the patient's energy for weight maintenance or gain. Option A is incorrect because the patient won't be able to participate effectively in talk therapy until she weighs at least 90 lb (40.8 kg). The nurse's verbally expressed concern (Option C) won't prevent further weight loss. Option D is inappropriate; the patient at this point is feeling out of control and requires much support and assistance.

44. Correct answer: C Negotiation gives the patient some responsibility for her continued treatment. Option A is premature; the patient may begin to lose weight again. Option B takes responsibility away from the patient. Option D is premature; psychotherapy may be indicated in the future, but it isn't the best intervention at this point.

45. Correct answer: C Careful observation is called for in this situation because you need to collect more data. Option A is incorrect because all patients shouldn't be punished for the actions of one or two and patients aren't responsible for the behavior of others. A unit-wide search (Option B) is premature at this point. Calling all the patients together (Option D) is a viable nursing action but has two drawbacks: some patients may interpret it as accusatory and it could alert the patient who's hiding the drug to be more careful.

46. Correct answer: B The patient is using a cognitive distortion that must be examined. Asking the patient to explain or clarify her conclusion focuses on the patient's thinking, or cognition. Options A and D focus instead on feelings. Option C focuses on the relationship rather than the thoughts behind the patient's statement.

47. Correct answer: A This is the only response that promotes personal growth because it makes the patient responsible for his own decision. Options B, C, and D place the nurse in a position of power over the patient.

48. Correct answer: D In the Gestalt mode, the patient would resolve unfinished business with her mother by "talking" to her. Option A represents a transactional analysis approach. Option B doesn't allow for self-discovery and isn't part of Gestalt theory. Option C is an approach used in cognitive theory.

49. Correct answer: B The patient has no concept of appropriate boundaries, indicating lack of differentiation, a key term in Sullivan's theory. Option A refers to one of the anxiety levels specified by Peplau. Option C refers to a developmental stage defined by Erikson. Option D reflects a Freudian approach.

50. Correct answer: D This response acknowledges and accepts the husband's anger and offers concrete information to clarify the misunderstanding. Options A and B are defensive communications. Option B also may block communication if the husband responds with no. Option C is a defensive restatement of the person's communication.

51. Correct answer: C Lithium alters sodium transport in nerve and muscle cells, slowing the speed of impulse transmission. Option A is incorrect because lithium has no known effect on body temperature. Option B is incorrect because lithium doesn't alter the transmission of pain impulses or cause lethargy. Renal failure (Option D) is a late sign of severe lithium toxicity.

52. Correct answer: C This response attempts to explore the patient's feelings. Options A and B assume that the patient is anxious (the nurse may be projecting feelings because of the patient's history of aggression). Option D ignores what might be going on with the patient.

53. Correct answer: B Although each option is an important area for assessment, a voluntary patient shouldn't be permitted to leave the hospital if dangerous to self or others.

54. Correct answer: D This response focuses on what may be the underlying need for which the delusion was created and it redirects the patient's attention to the current, reality-based situation. Options A, B, and C don't assist the patient in giving up the delusion; in fact, they reinforce it.

55. Correct answer: C This response provides a structure for reducing the patient's anxiety, gaining insight into his behavior and, eventually, redirecting his anxiety. Options A, B, and D don't assist the patient in gaining insight into his behavior and may increase his anxiety.

56. Correct answer: D This response acknowledges the patient's feelings and conveys the nurse's ability to understand them. Options A and C promote a negative self-image rather than attempting to enhance the patient's self-esteem. Option B dismisses the patient's current feelings.

57. Correct answer: C This response acknowledges the patient's behavior and asks the patient to provide further information about why she's seeking help. Options A and D don't address the reason the patient is seeking help. Option B doesn't respond to the patient's plea for help.

58. Correct answer: C This response indicates that the patient's feelings are okay and that you're comfortable with how he feels. Options A and B imply that the patient's feelings aren't legitimate. Option D evades the issue and only relieves the nurse's anxiety, not the patient's.

59. Correct answer: C This response enables you to collect more information from the patient. Options A and B cut off the discussion. Option D is too specific and may inhibit the patient from elaborating further.

60. Correct answer: C Having the patient help with laundry rechannels his energy in a positive activity. Option A doesn't take into account that the patient needs direction and structure, not seclusion. Option B ignores the patient's impaired judgment and poor impulse control. Option D doesn't assist the patient in controlling the behavior.

Analyzing the posttest

Total the number of *incorrect* responses to the posttest. A score of 1 to 9 indicates that you have an excellent knowledge base and are well prepared for the certification examination; a score of 10 to 14 indicates adequate preparation, although more study or improvement in test-taking skills is recommended; a score of 15 or more indicates the need for intensive study before taking the certification examination.

For a more detailed analysis of your performance, complete the self-diagnostic profile on page 264.

Posttest self-diagnostic profile

In the top row of boxes, record the number of each question you answered incorrectly. Then, beneath each question number, check the box that corresponds to the reason you answered the question incorrectly, along with the category of client need and nursing process for that question. Finally, tabulate the number of check marks on each line in the right-hand column marked "Totals." You now have an individualized profile of weak areas that require further study or improvement in test-taking ability before you take the Psychiatric and Mental Health Nursing Certification Examination.

Question number																					Totals
Test-taking skills																					
1. Misread question																					
2. Missed important point																					
3. Forgot fact or concept																					
4. Applied wrong fact or concept																					
5. Drew wrong conclusion																					
6. Incorrectly evaluated distracters																					
7. Mistakenly filled in wrong answer																					
8. Read into question																					
9. Guessed wrong																					
10. Misunderstood question																					
Client need																					
1. Safe, effective care environment																					
2. Physiologic integrity																					
3. Psychosocial integrity																					
4. Health promotion and maintenance																					
Nursing process																					
1. Assessment																					
2. Analysis																					
3. Planning																					
4. Implementation																					
5. Evaluation																					

Selected references

Carson, V.B. *Mental Health Nursing: The Nurse-Patient Journey*, 2nd ed. Philadelphia: W.B. Saunders Co., 2000.

Cummings, J.L., et al. "Efficacy of Metrifonate in Improving the Psychiatric and Behavioral Disturbances of Patients with Alzheimer's Disease," *Journal of Geriatric Psychiatry and Neurology* 14(2):101-8, Summer 2001.

DeBattista, C., and Mueller, K. "Is Electroconvulsive Therapy Effective for the Depressed Patient with Comorbid Borderline Personality Disorder?" *Journal of Electroconvulsive Therapy* 17(2):91-98, June 2001.

Diagnostic and Statistical Manual of Mental Disorders, 4th ed., Text Revision (*DSM-IV-TR*). Washington, D.C.: American Psychiatric Association, 2000.

Fishel, A.H. "Nursing Management of Anxiety and Panic," *Nursing Clinics of North America* 33(1):135-51, March 1998.

Fontaine, K.L., and Fletcher, J.S. *Mental Health Nursing*, 4th ed. Menlo Park, Ca.: Addison-Wesley, 1999.

Fortinash, K., and Holoday-Worret, P. *Psychiatric Mental Health Nursing*, 2nd ed. St. Louis: Mosby–Year Book, Inc., 2000.

Gabbard, G.O., et al. *Treatments of Psychiatric Disorders*, 3rd ed. Washington, D.C.: American Psychiatric Press, 2001.

Haber, J., et al. *Comprehensive Psychiatric Nursing*, 5th ed. St. Louis: Mosby–Year Book, Inc., 1997.

Katon, W., et al. "Medical Symptoms without Identified Pathology; Related to Psychiatric Disorders, Childhood and Adult Trauma and Personality Traits," *Annals of Internal Medicine* 134 (9 Pt 2):917-25, May 2001.

Martenyi, F., et al. "Gender Differences in the Efficacy of Fluoxetine and Maprotiline in Depressed Patients: A Double-blind Trial of Antidepressants with Serotonergic or Norepinephrine Reuptake Inhibition Profile," *European Neuropsychopharmacology* 11(3):227-32, June 2001.

Martin, S.D., et al. "Brain Blood Flow Changes in Depressed Patients Treated with Interpersonal Psychotherapy or Venlafaxine Hydrochloride: Preliminary Findings," *Archives of General Psychiatry* 58(7):641-48, July 2001.

Morrow, L.A., et al. "Neuropsychological Assessment, Depression and Past Exposure to Organic Solvents," *Applied Neuropsychology* 8(2):65-73, 2001.

Rogers, A., et al. "Experiencing Depression, Experiencing the Depressed: The Separate Worlds of Patients and Doctors," *Journal of Mental Health* 10(3):317-33, 2001.

Schatzberg, A.F., and Nemeroff, C.B. *The American Psychiatric Press Textbook of Psychopharmacology*, 2nd ed. Washington, D.C.: American Psychiatric Press, 1998.

Snowdon, J. "Later-Life Depression: What Can Be Done?" *Australian Prescriber* 24(3):65-67, 2001.

Stuart, G., and Laraia, M. *Principles and Practice of Psychiatric Nursing,* 7th ed. St. Louis: Mosby–Year Book, Inc., 2001.

Townsend, M. *Mental Health Nursing: Concepts of Care,* 3rd ed. Philadelphia: F.A. Davis Co., 2000.

Woodward, B. "Improving Adherence to Psychiatric Medication: Office-based Approaches," *Psychiatric Times* Vol. XVII, Issue 6, June 2001. *www.mhsource.com/pt/p010649.html*

Index

t refers to a table.

t refers to a table.

Certification examination, 1-6
  eligibility and application for, 1-2, 2t
  preparing for, 4-5
  test plan for, 3
  test-taking strategies for, 5-6, 6t
Child protection laws, 79
Childhood, developmental characteristics of, 22, 23
Children, and play therapy, 193
Children Are People, 103
Chloral hydrate, 215t
Chloral hydrate derivatives, 214, 215t
Chlordiazepoxide, 213t, 217
Chlorpromazine, 198, 202t
Chromosome 6, and schizophrenia, 166
Clarification, in crisis intervention, 15
Clichés, in therapeutic communication, 63, 67
Clinical nurse specialist, 34
Clonazepam, 213t
Clorazepate, 213t
Clozapine, 203t
Clozaril, 203t
Cocaine, 99t, 102, 111
Cocaine Anonymous, 103
Code for Nurses with Interpretive Statements, 69
Cogentin, 206t
Cognitive approach, 251, 261
Cognitive development, stages of, 21
Collaboration, standards of psychiatric and mental health clinical nursing practice and, 234
Collegiality, standards of psychiatric and mental health clinical nursing practice and, 233
Commitment
  involuntary, 72, 73
  voluntary, 72, 253, 262
Common law, 70
Communication, 245, 257
  ego, 187
  in family therapy, 192
  privileged, 77
  therapeutic. See Therapeutic communication.
  types of, 61
  Watzlawick's pragmatics of, 47
Communication disturbance, in schizophrenia, 168
Communication model, of behavior, 47, 51

Community health center, nurse's role in, 37
Community Mental Health Centers Act, 198
Compensation, as coping mechanism, 13
Compulsions, 85t
Confidentiality
  breach of, 69
  patient rights and, 77
Confinement, legal aspects of, 72-75
Confrontation, as communication technique, 64
Constipation, psychotropic drugs and, 200t
Constitutional law, 70
Consultation, standards of psychiatric and mental health clinical nursing practice and, 229
Conversion, as coping mechanism, 13
Conversion disorder, 178-179, 182-183
  diagnostic criteria for, 177
  management of, 184, 185, 245, 249, 257, 259
Coping, 12-13
Counseling, 225
Countertransference, 13-14, 187
Crack, 99t
Crisis, 14-16
Crisis intervention, 15
Cyclothymic disorder, 136

D

Dalmane, 213t
Defense mechanisms
  in crisis intervention, 15
  ego-centered, 12, 13
Deinstitutionalization Movement, 199
Delirium, 142-144, 146-147, 148
  diagnostic criteria for, 143
Delirium substance withdrawal, 97
Delusional thinking, 174, 243, 256
Delusions, management of, 245, 257
Dementia, 144-145, 147, 148
  diagnostic criteria for, 143
  management of, 145, 149
Denial, as coping mechanism, 13
Dependent personality disorder, 154, 160
Depersonalization disorder, 123t, 126-127, 130

t refers to a table.

Genuineness, as communication technique, 62, 66
Gestalt therapy, 186, 196, 252, 261
Graded exposure, 189
Grief, 11-12
  stages of, 11, 17
Grindler's neurolinguistic programming, 47
Grounded theory, in nursing research, 58
Group therapy, 190-193, 197
  in addiction disorders, 105
  management of, 247, 248, 258, 259

H
Halazepam, 213t
Halcion, 213t
Haldol, 202t, 216
Halfway house, 104
Hallucinations, in schizophrenia, 172, 174
Hallucinogens, 99t
Haloperidol, 202t, 216
Health Care and Political Agenda for Change, 32
Health promotion and maintenance, 228
Health teaching, standards of psychiatric and mental health clinical nursing practice and, 227
Hematologic system, effects of alcohol abuse on, 100
Heroin, 98t
Histrionic personality disorder, 153, 158
Human development, 18-26
  cognitive and moral models of, 20-21
  interpersonal models of, 21-22
  life cycle characteristics of, 22-24
  psychoanalytic models of, 18-20, 39
Human Rights Guidelines for Nurses in Clinical and Other Research, 53
Humanistic model, of behavior, 48-49
Hydroxyzine, 215t
Hypertensive crisis, 210, 246, 250, 258, 260
Hypochondriasis, 179-180, 184, 185
  diagnostic criteria for, 177
Hypomania, 244, 256
Hypotension, 150, 260
Hypothesis, in nursing research, 56, 60

I
Id, 18, 38
Identification, as coping mechanism, 13
"I" message, 243, 256
Imipramine, 208t
IMPROVE, 32
Infancy, developmental characteristics of, 22
Influenza virus, and schizophrenia, 167
Informed consent, 70-72
Intellectualization, as coping mechanism, 13
Interpersonal development, stages of, 21
Interpersonal model, of behavior, 41-43
Interpersonal theory, of depression, 132
Interpersonal therapy, 46
Intoxication, nursing management of, 98-99t
Invasion of privacy, 69
Irrational belief, 188

J
Janimine, 208t
Jaundice, psychotropic drugs and, 200t
Joint Commission on Accreditation of Healthcare Organizations, 31

K
Kava-kava, 17
Klonopin, 213t
Kohlberg, moral development theory of, 21, 26

L
La belle indifference, 178, 182
Language disturbance, in schizophrenia, 168
Leadership, mental health team and, 30, 36
Legal aspects of nursing, 68-80
  assault and battery and, 75-76
  child protection laws and, 79
  confinement and, 72-75
  documentation of care and, 78-79
  informed consent and, 70-72
  patient rights and, 76-78
  torts and, 68-70
Lewin, behavioral theory of, 49
Libido, changes in, psychotropic drugs and, 200t
Librium, 213t, 217

t refers to a table.

---

t refers to a table.

---

t refers to a table.